OXFORD MEDICAL PUBLICATIONS

Oxford Handbook of
ENT and
Head and Neck
Surgery

Published and forthcoming Oxford Handbooks

WV 100

Oxford Handbook of ENT and Head and Neck Surgery

SECOND EDITION

Rogan Corbridge

Clinical Tutor and ENT Consultant,
Royal Berkshire Hospital,
Reading, and
Programme Director and Consultant ENT Surgeon,
John Radcliffe Hospital,
Oxford, UK

Nicholas Steventon

Consultant ENT Surgeon,
Taranaki Base Hospital,
New Plymouth,
New Zealand

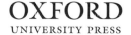

OXFORD
UNIVERSITY PRESS

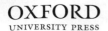

OXFORD
UNIVERSITY PRESS

Great Clarendon Street, Oxford OX2 6DP

Oxford University Press is a department of the University of Oxford.
It furthers the University's objective of excellence in research, scholarship,
and education by publishing worldwide in

Oxford New York

Auckland Cape Town Dar es Salaam Hong Kong Karachi
Kuala Lumpur Madrid Melbourne Mexico City Nairobi
New Delhi Shanghai Taipei Toronto

With offices in

Argentina Austria Brazil Chile Czech Republic France Greece
Guatemala Hungary Italy Japan Poland Portugal Singapore
South Korea Switzerland Thailand Turkey Ukraine Vietnam

Oxford is a registered trade mark of Oxford University Press
in the UK and in certain other countries

Published in the United States
by Oxford University Press Inc., New York

British Library Cataloguing in Publication Data
Data available

Library of Congress Cataloging-in-Publication-Data
Data available

Typeset by Cepha Imaging Private Ltd, Bangalore, India
Printed in China
on acid-free paper by
Asia Pacific Offset

ISBN 978–0–19–9550791

10 9 8 7 6 5 4 3 2 1

Contents

Detailed contents

Overview

Using this book

The aim of this book, like all the other Oxford Handbooks, is to provide a compact but comprehensive guide to medical practice. It has been designed to slip inside the pocket of a white coat and to be rapidly retrieved for reference. There are many blank facing pages for notes, and for amending or annotating the text to fit in with local practice.

The core text is based on an anatomical list of ear nose and throat diseases. There are separate sections on ENT examinations, investigations, common operations, ward care, and emergencies. There is also a separate section on the work of other ENT health professionals.

Chapter 3, 'Common methods of presentation', is unique for this type of book. This chapter is a guide for dealing with patients as they present in clinical practice. It also provides a convenient way of accessing the relevant chapter in the anatomical list.

We hope that the book will be well used and will help guide you through the sometimes complex world of ENT.

ENT as a subject and career

ENT is a fantastic ... theory. It is difficult t... diversity in medical prac...

- ENT conditions make up ... every bit as exciting in practice as it is in any specialty which can provide such
- ENT conditions affect peop...
- Outpatient work is about 50% ... ll general practice consultations. balance between surgical and med... from neonates to the elderly. the body to major head and neck recons... workload. This gives a good
- ENT is an expanding surgical specialty that i... the smallest bones in general surgery in areas such as parotid surgery... surgery.
- Cosmetic surgery is undertaken in ENT, in the for... over traditional thyroid surgery.
- Surgery is also performed on the skull base and pituitary gland. facial plstics.
- ENT offers enormous research potential, from nasal polyps to congenital hearing loss.
- There are cutting edge developments occurring in ENT, such as cochlear implantation.

We hope that your experiences in ENT will fill you with enthusiasm for this specialty.

Further sources of information

ENT UK website: ✍ www.entuk.org
Royal College of Surgeons website: ✍ www.rcseng.ac.uk

Student ENT

The subject of ENT can seem qui͏. ͏s students. Particularly as this vast subject occupies such a ͏ ͏he curriculum, and has been dropped entirely from some m͏ ͏s.

In strong contrast to the ͏ to it in training, ENT conditions make up between 25 and ͏ general practice consultations. As a student, it is important ͏ a firm idea in your mind of important topics you want to cove͏ ͏. These will form your learning aims and objectives—see the lis͏ site. There may be local variations.

You will find th͏T departments throughout the world are welcoming to stud͏but do not abuse their hospitality by being late or discourteous. Pro͏onal conduct is important whatever specialty you are studyng.

There are pa͏cularly sensitive areas within ENT practice which require special tact as a student. Two of these are:

Head and neck cancer

These cancers form a large part of the ENT workload. You will need to be sensitive in dealing with these patients. They often have unique problems associated with their disease and treatment. These may include:

- Poor communication
- Disfiguring surgery
- Depression
- Alcohol withdrawal

Hearing problems

The diagnosis of hearing loss in a child can be a devastating blow to parents. You will need to be sensitive to this. Another cause of great concern to parents is when a poorly performing child has a normal hearing test, as this may confirm the diagnosis of global developmental delay.

ENT learning aims and objectives for clinical medical students

Aims

- To acquire sufficient knowledge of ENT conditions to be able to recognize common problems and when and what to refer.
- To understand that ENT conditions are extremely common and form a large part of the workload of a general practitioner.
- To learn the skills required to examine patients with ENT diseases and to make a presumptive diagnosis.
- To learn how to prioritize and manage different ENT conditions.
- To become stimulated and interested in the specialty of ENT.

Objectives

- To learn the signs and symptoms of common ENT conditions.
- To learn the techniques of ear, nasal, and neck examination.
- To demonstrate an understanding of the basic anatomy and physiology of the ear and upper aerodigestive tract, and relate this knowledge to the signs and symptoms of ENT disease.
- To understand the medical and surgical treatment of common ENT conditions.
- To be familiar with the commonly used medications for treating ENT problems, and their side effects.
- To understand the risks and complications of surgery.
- To recognize the different ways in which head and neck malignancy can present, and to understand that early diagnosis of head and neck cancer leads to improved survival.
- To learn the ways in which ENT-related communication difficulties can arise and be overcome.
- To appreciate and be sensitive to the impact of ENT conditions on patients and their families.

Student ENT curriculum

Practical skills
- Use of the auriscope to examine the external auditory meatus and tympanic membrane
- Basic examination of the nose
- Examination of the oral cavity and oropharynx
- Examination of the neck
- How to manage a nosebleed
- How to deal with a tracheostomy

Ear
- Basic anatomy and physiology of the ear
- Presentation and management of common ear disease, e.g. otitis externa, otitis media, glue ear, chronic suppurative otitis media (cholesteatoma), vertigo, and facial palsy
- Examination of the ear, including the pinna, ear canal, and otoscopy
- Testing the hearing with tuning fork tests
- The advantages of the microscope and the fibreoptic otoscope
- Basic interpretation of play audiometry, pure tone audiograms, and tympanograms
- The principles of grommet insertion, mastoid surgery, and the treatment of Ménière's disease
- Identifying postoperative problems following ear surgery, i.e. sensorineural hearing loss, facial nerve palsy, and vestibular dysfunction
- Understanding the differential diagnosis of facial nerve palsy and its treatment

Nose
- Anatomy and physiology of the nose
- Symptoms and signs of common sinonasal disease, e.g. rhinitis, sinusitis, nasal polyps
- Examination of the nose, including an assessment of the appearance, the septum, the turbinates, and the mucosa
- The endoscopic evaluation of the nose
- Management of a fractured nose and the timing of intervention
- Management of epistaxis, from minor nosebleeds to torrential haemorrhage
- The principles of common nasal operations, including septal surgery, functional endoscopic sinus surgery, and rhinoplasty

Head and neck—benign and malignant disease

- The basic anatomy and physiology of the oral cavity, salivary glands, pharynx, larynx, oesophagus, and lymph node drainage
- The presentation of head and neck cancer
- The presentation and management of salivary gland disease
- Examining the oral cavity, larynx, and pharynx, including the use of the nasendoscope
- Examining the neck with reference to the lymph nodes
- The role of fine needle aspiration cytology
- The principles and limitations of radiological investigation of the head and neck region
- Management of neck lumps, in particular the malignant lymph node with an unknown primary
- The management of the airway in patients with a tracheostomy or end tracheostomy after laryngectomy
- A basic knowledge of the principles of operative surgery, in particular the principles of reconstructive surgery and the surgery for salivary gland disease, e.g. parotidectomy
- The postoperative management of a patient who has undergone major head and neck surgery
- The role of the multidisciplinary team in head and neck cancer and voice disorders

Supplementary knowledge

- The role of otoacoustic emissions and evoked auditory potentials in managing hearing loss
- The use of speech audiometry
- The surgery for otosclerosis
- Bone-anchored hearing aids for conductive hearing loss
- Cochlear implantation and the reactions of the deaf community to this intervention
- The use of sign language
- Neuro-otology, in particular the presentation and management of acoustic neuromas
- Craniofacial surgery and the interplay between ENT, plastic surgery, and neurosurgery
- The management of cleft palate and the increased risk of glue ear
- Advanced endoscopic sinus surgery for the management of sinonasal malignancy, pituitary tumours, and skull base tumours
- Microlaryngeal surgery and surgical voice restoration
- The use of chemotherapy and radiotherapy in head and neck malignancy

Research

Make this a priority in your mind. It is important to keep your CV moving and improving. Aim to produce at least one publication every six months. Don't be distracted by trying to be involved in too many projects at once.

Work in a team if you can, to maximize your publications. Don't take on too many projects in a team—each team member should take on one research project at a time. Ask senior colleagues about possible projects, and affiliated university departments may be helpful. Involve a statistician before undertaking research. This will often help turn an idea into a first-rate publication and avoid unnecessary work. Always check local ethics committee guidelines before you start.

Research is expected but not everyone needs to produce a D. Phil.

Minimum requirements for entry into specialist training:
• One publication in a peer-reviewed journal
• Three presentations at national meetings
• Full understanding of research methods, including statistical interpretation
• Critical appraisal skills to evaluate published material

Audit

Audit is often regarded as a poor relative of research. At its best, audit can be very informative and can lead to changes in practice.

Involvement in audit is an expected part of professional practice. There are many opportunities available and help is often on hand from audit departments within the hospital.

Like research, make sure that you plan an audit that will achieve something with a tangible result. The best audits provide a completion of the audit cycle (📖 see Fig. 1.1).

Types of audit
• Structure—how the system is set up
• Process—how the system works
• Outcome—the product of the system
• Departmental—audits which are carried out in your department
• Regional—audits carried out in your region
• National—audits carried out by national organizations, such as the National Tonsillectomy Audit, NCEPOD

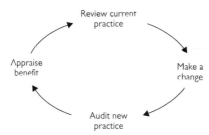

Fig. 1.1 The audit cycle diagram.

The ENT examination

Equipment

A fully equipped ENT department will have all the necessary instruments for performing a full ENT examination. However, if you are a GP, or if you are working in another specialty, you will need to obtain a basic equipment kit.

ENT SHOs or SpRs will also need to have such a kit when visiting patients at home or visiting peripheral hospitals.

Basic equipment

- A light source—a portable headlight that runs off batteries is ideal
- Wooden tongue depressors
- Thudicum speculum
- An otoscope with several speculae
- Pneumatic attachment for the otoscope
- Tuning fork 512Hz
- Pen and paper
- Gloves

Advanced equipment

- Lidocaine 5%/phenylphrine 0.5% (lidocaine with phenylephrine) spray for decongesting and anaesthetizing the nose
- A flexible nasendoscope with light source
- Alcohol skin swabs to act as demister for the scope
- Water-based gel to lubricate the scope

Emergency equipment

- Large nasal tampons, e.g. Merocel® (you can always cut 10cm ones to size)
- Silver nitrate sticks
- Foley-type urinary catheters (to control posterior epistaxis)

On-call tip

Many SpRs are not resident on-call. Therefore always pack an emergency kit box to leave in your car. This can be passed from SpR to SpR nightly. Even some of the most basic pieces of equipment are sometimes impossible to find in the middle of the night.

Examination of the ear

The examination should be practised and repeated regularly so that it becomes routine. It is equally important to document the findings of any examination accurately.

Routine examination

- Ask the patient which is their better hearing ear and start by examining this ear.
- Check with the patient that their ear is not painful.
- Examine the pinna and look for preauricular abnormalities.
- Examine for surgical scars in front of and behind the pinna. Also examine the hairline above the pinna (📖 see Fig. 2.1).
- Straighten the external ear canal (EAC) by pulling the pinna up and backwards (if you are examining a baby pull backwards only).
- Examine the EAC skin and document any changes using an otoscope.
- Clean any debris from the EAC using a microscope and suction clearance as required. It is very important to remove debris from the tympanic membrane, which may be obscuring serious disease. Be gentle as this can be uncomfortable.
- Systematically examine the tympanic membrane. You cannot see all the eardrum at once with a standard otoscope. It needs to be looked at in segments due to a limited field of view through the speculum.
- First visualize the handle of the malleus and follow it up to the lateral process. Then you will not miss the superior part of the drum. You may need to kneel down to get the correct angle.
- Perform pneumatic otoscopy.
- Repeat with the pathological ear.
- Perform tuning fork tests (📖 see p. 17).
- Perform a free field test of hearing (📖 see p. 20).
- Check facial nerve function (📖 see 'Facial nerve palsy', p. 378).
- Visualize the postnasal space with an endoscope or mirror.
- Perform an otoneurological examination if the patient has symptoms of vestibular dysfunction or you suspect vestibular dysfunction from the observed pathology.

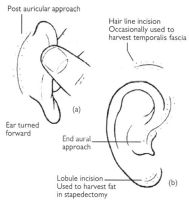

Fig. 2.1 Common ear incisions.

Know your otoscope

Each type of otoscope is turned on in a slightly different way—although usually by twisting it at the top of the body. Nothing inspires less confidence when you are examining a patient than being unable to turn on the otoscope. It should be held like a pen with the little finger extended—like an affected tea drinker—to touch the patient's cheek. This enables an early warning of head-turning particularly in children. The right hand holds the otoscope for the right ear examination and vice versa. 📖 See Fig. 2.2.

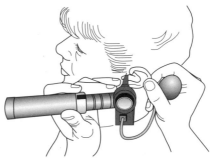

Fig. 2.2 Otoscopy with pneumatic bulb.

How to perform pneumatic otoscopy

- Hold the pinna and otoscope as when performing standard otoscopy. The only difference is that the insufflator bulb is held in the hand retracting the pinna. This feels slightly awkward initially but becomes easier with practice.
- Use a special speculum with a soft tip so that a tight seal is formed by the speculum in the outer part of the EAC.
- Whilst viewing the centre of the tympanic membrane squeeze the insufflator bulb. Under normal circumstances and with a tight seal the tympanic membrane is displaced away from the observer by the application of positive pressure.
- When the insufflator bulb is released this causes a negative pressure and the normal tympanic membrane will move outwards.

Tuning fork tests

These are simple tests of hearing which are most often used to differentiate between a conductive and a sensorineural hearing loss.

They should be performed with a 512Hz tuning fork. If the frequency is lower, then vibrations are produced which can mislead patients who think this is an auditory stimulus.

The ends of a tuning fork are known as tines not prongs. The loudest sound from the tuning fork is produced at the end of the tine. The tine moves a greater distance at the tip displacing more air and hence producing a louder sound.

Start the tuning fork by hitting your elbow or knee with it. Plucking the tines produces less efficient sound and hitting a table or desk edge produces overtones.

Weber's and Rinne's tests are performed together as a 'package' to help identify the type of hearing loss.

Weber's tuning fork test

In normal hearing, sound is not localized to either ear. In sensorineural hearing loss the non-affected ear hears the sound loudest. In conductive loss the sound is heard loudest in the affected ear.

In this test, the tuning fork is placed at the top of the patient's head (Fig. 2.3). The patient then says which ear hears the sound loudest, or if it is in the middle.

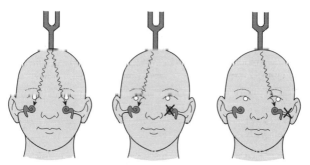

Fig. 2.3 Diagrams of tuning fork tests.

Rinne's test

This test compares air conduction with bone conduction. The activated tuning fork is placed behind the patient's ear, against the mastoid process (Fig. 2.4). The patient is asked to say when they stop hearing the stimulus. The tuning fork is then moved to a position 2cm away from the external auditory meatus (EAM) and held with the tips of the tines level and in line with the ear canal. The patient is then asked if they can hear the sound.

This test can be modified by moving the tuning fork from the mastoid to the EAM before the sound has diminished. The patient is then asked which is the loudest sound.

These test results can be confusing, because a pathological test result is called a negative test! This is contrary to almost all other tests in medicine where a positive result is an abnormal result and a negative result is normal.

- *Positive test*: air conduction is better than bone conduction.
- *Negative test*: bone conduction is better than air conduction.

> **False-negative Rinne's test**
>
> This happens when the sound is actually being heard by the other ear. Sound conducted by bone is absorbed and travels across the skull, so when the tuning fork is placed on the left side it will be heard almost as well by the right inner ear as the left. To stop this effect the other ear can be masked.

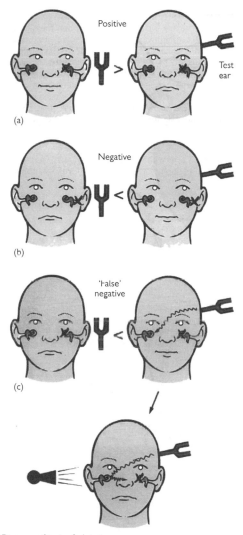

Fig. 2.4 Diagrams of tuning fork tests.

Free field test of hearing

Patients will usually have a formal audiogram when they attend an ENT outpatients appointment. However, there are some situations when you may need to make a rough guess at a patient's hearing threshold. This might happen because there are no formal audiometric facilities available, or if you suspect a patient may be exaggerating a hearing loss.

During this test, your own voice is used as a sound stimulus, while the patient's non-test ear is masked by rubbing your finger over the tragus. This produces some sound, which helps to 'mask' that ear. Practice is essential as the positioning for this procedure can be awkward ([ ] see Fig. 2.5).

Procedure

- Shield the patient's eyes with your hand.
- Rub the tragus of the non-test ear with your forefinger to mask the sound in this ear.
- Whisper a number at approximately 60cm from the test ear.
- If the patient cannot hear, use a normal-volume spoken voice, followed by a shout if necessary.
- Repeat with opposite ear.

Patients should be 50% accurate at repeating your words to pass the test. If they hear your whisper at a distance of 60cm, then their hearing is better than 30dB.

Examining tip

You can perform a cruder version of this test in a covert manner. When the patient sits in front of you, a whispered question as you hold the patient's notes in front of your mouth can produce an interesting response, not always corresponding to the patient's seemingly poor audiogram!

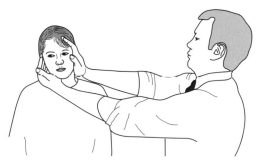

Fig. 2.5 Positioning for free field testing.

Otoneurological examination

The inner ear is an integral part of the balance system. It is important to evaluate the balance system and be competent at performing a neurological examination.

Remember—when dealing with ENT disease:

- The disease itself can produce neurological disturbance
- Complications of the disease can cause neurological problems
- Other neurological problems can mimic ENT disease

The examination should include:

- Cranial nerve examination
- Assessment of tone, power, co-ordination, and sensation of the limbs, trunk, and neck

Special ENT neurological tests

- Romberg's
- Dix–Hallpike test
- Unterburger's test
- Nystagmus
  - 1st degree
  - 2nd degree
  - 3rd degree
- Facial nerve evaluation
  - acoustic reflexes
  - Schirmer's test

Examination of the nose

The most difficult part of this examination is learning to hold the Thudicum's speculum. This is a bit like a nose clip used in swimming but in reverse—it holds the nose open rather than closed.

Basic position

The patient should be sitting in a swivel chair opposite the seated examiner. It is useful to have the patient's chair slightly higher than the examiner's chair. A good light source is essential: either a bull lamp positioned over the patient's left shoulder reflected onto your head mirror and back at the patient; alternatively, and preferably on the ward, use a headlight. Keep your legs together and place them alongside and parallel to the patient's legs. This allows you to get less than an arm's length away from the patient to examine and perform any necessary procedures.

Examination is systematic as always.

External nose

- Check for scars.
- Look at the skin type and thickness.
- Observe and palpate the nasal bones, upper lateral and lower lateral cartilages.
- Look for symmetry and abnormal seating of the cartilages with the patient in the right and left lateral position and straight on.
- Tilt the head back to view the columella and alar cartilages in a similar way.

Internal nose

- Check the patency of each nasal airway.
- Occlude one nostril with a thumb and then ask the patient to sniff in through their nose.
- Repeat on the opposite side.
- In children, a metal tongue depressor held under the nose will show exhaled air; if there is a blockage, if will not steam up.
- If there is an obstruction and the nostril collapses perform Cottle's test (Fig. 2.6). Lateral pressure on the skin of the cheek lateral to the nose can stop nasal collapse if there is obstruction at the nasal valve. Alternatively, a probe such as a Jobson–Horne can be inserted into the nose. Tenting the nostril at various positions can stop the collapse and further localize a site of weakness.
- Inspect the nose internally using Thudicum's speculum. An otoscope with a large speculum can be used for children who don't like the bright headlight or the Thudicums.
- Assess the straightness and integrity of the septum.
- Assess the size of the turbinates.
- Note the mucosal appearance.
- Use the endoscope to assess the posterior part of the nose.
- Feel for lymph nodes.

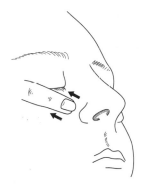

Fig. 2.6 Cottle's test.

Postnasal space examination (Fig. 2.7)

- Inspect the posterior choanae and postnasal space with an endoscope or with a mirror.
- Anaesthetize the oropharynx with lidocaine 5%/phenylephrine 0.5% (lidocaine with phenylephrine).
- Hold a Luc's tongue depressor in your right hand and use it to depress the patient's tongue
- With your other hand, run a small mirror along the top of the tongue depressor to enter the oropharynx behind the soft palate.
- The reflected light should illuminate the postnasal space to visualize the posterior choanae and the ends of the inferior turbinates. Any adenoidal tissue will also be seen

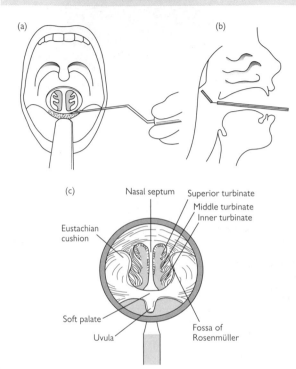

Fig. 2.7 Visualization of postnasal space (PNS).

Endoscopic examination

Rigid and flexible endoscopes can be used to visualize the tympanic membranes, nasal cavity, and the laryngeal–pharyngeal areas. Video cameras and still cameras can be attached to the scopes to provide real-time visualization on TV monitors and allow recording for documentation purposes. This can make explanations of pathology easier for the patient to understand in areas that are not normally visualized.

Otoendoscopy

A short 4mm or 2.7mm rigid endoscope can be used to visualize the tympanic membrane and EAC. The wide viewing angle provides a view of the whole tympanic membrane. It can be performed without local anaesthesia. Inserting a speculum of a standard otoscope into the EAC can help stop the endoscope touching the walls of the EAC, which can be painful. The scope can be passed straight through the speculum.

Rigid and flexible nasendoscopy

- Sit the patient in a chair with a headrest (a parent or relative can help support the head if the headrest is unsuitable). Lying the patient down on an examination couch with their head slightly flexed by resting on a pillow can also be useful for rigid endoscopy. It is similar to the operating position.
- Before starting, warn the patient that the nasal spray tastes dreadful, that their throat will be numb and that hot food or drink should not be consumed for an hour to avoid burns.

Preparation of the nose

- Prepare the patient's nose with lidocaine with phenylephrine spray—usually five sprays to each nostril. The anaesthetic and vasoconstrictive effect of the spray takes 6 minutes to work. So it is essential to wait 6 minutes before starting the procedure. A diluted solution of lidocaine with phenylephrine can be given to children.
- Patients will still feel the movement of the scope. Some areas of the nose may require further topical application of local anaesthesia during the procedure—use cotton wool soaked in lidocaine with phenylephrine and apply using a Tilley's nasal dressing forceps.

Rigid nasal endoscopy

- Prepare the nose as above.
- Two 4mm rigid Hopkins' rods of 0° and 30° viewing angles are used to provide the best view of the nose. Sometimes 2.7mm diameter scopes are used either in the narrow nose or the child's nose.
- The nose is systematically examined using a three-pass technique (Figs 2.8–2.10).

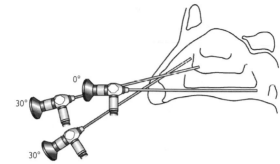

Fig. 2.8 Three-pass technique.

1) View along floor of nose to postnasal space

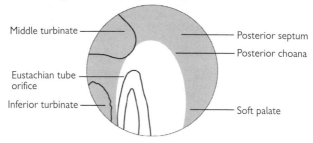

Middle turbinate — Posterior septum
— Posterior choana

Eustachian tube orifice

Inferior turbinate — Soft palate

2) View into middle meatus

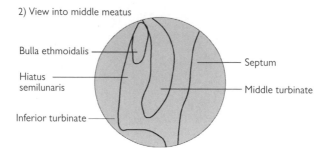

Bulla ethmoidalis — Septum

Hiatus semilunaris — Middle turbinate

Inferior turbinate —

3) View into frontal recess

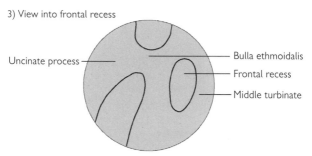

Uncinate process — Bulla ethmoidalis
— Frontal recess
— Middle turbinate

Fig. 2.9 Views on endoscopy seen during the three passes.

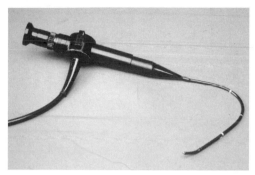

Fig. 2.10 Nasendoscope and controls.

Flexible nasal endoscopy
- Prepare the nose.
- Lubricate the scope with water-soluble gel.
- Wipe the end of the scope with an alcohol swab. This prevents it misting up in the warm nose.
- Hold the scope controls with your dominant hand and support the tip with your other hand. View the alcohol swab's packet or the text on the local anaesthetic bottle to check for focus. Make sure you are happy with the scope's direction of movement when you operate the controls. Nasopharyngoscopes can only be actively moved up or down using the controls, but rotation of the whole scope can produce a degree of lateral movement.
- Begin by feeding the scope a few centimetres into the nose using your non-dominant hand. Visualize the nasal cavity as you do this.
- The scope should pass above the inferior turbinate and below the middle turbinate. Try to keep the scope parallel to the upper surface of the inferior turbinate. Use the up–down control sparingly at this point to keep the scope straight. Advance the scope until the posterior choana and Eustachian tube orifice are visualized.
- Ask the patient to swallow—the Eustachian tube will be observed; the palate will also move.
- Direct the scope end-downwards and advance it to visualize the larynx. Patients can be asked to swallow to find the way and this can also clean the end of the scope if mucus obscures the view.
- When the larynx is visualized, ask the patient to:
  - breathe in and out quietly
  - take a deep breath
  - say 'eeee'—a single tone.
- During this time assess the movement of the vocal cords, their structure and function.

Stroboscopy can also be used to provide further details of the vocal cord function.

Common methods of presentation

Hoarse voice

History	Examination	Diagnosis	📖 Page no.
Lasted less than 2 weeks + pyrexia + a sore throat + URTI symptoms	⟶ Acute laryngitis		220
Lasted more than 3 weeks Constant Progressive Patient is a smoker ± dysphagia ± pain ± otalgia ± a neck lump	⟶ Vocal cord lesion ⟶ Unilateral	Laryngeal cancer Vocal polyp Vocal granuloma Papillomata	224 230 230 230
	⟶ Bilateral	Reinke's oedema Papillomata Singer's nodules	221 230 230
	⟶ Immobile	Vocal cord palsy	231
Variable + voice abuse Comes and goes ± GORD	⟶ No vocal cord lesion	Muscle tension dysphonia	231

Epistaxis (nosebleed)

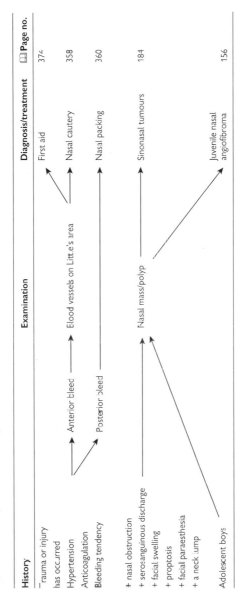

History	Examination	Diagnosis/treatment	📖 Page no.
Trauma or injury has occurred	→ Anterior bleed → Blood vessels on Little's area →	First aid	374
Hypertension		Nasal cautery	358
Anticoagulation			
Bleeding tendency	→ Posterior bleed →	Nasal packing	360
+ nasal obstruction			
+ serosanguinous discharge	→ Nasal mass/polyp →	Sinonasal tumours	184
+ facial swelling			
+ proptosis			
+ facial paraesthesia			
+ a neck lump			
Adolescent boys	→	Juvenile nasal angiofibroma	156

Dysphagia (swallowing difficulty)

History	Examination	Diagnosis	📖 Page no.
Constant	⟶ a neck lump	Carcinoma	256
Progressive	Endoscopy—lesion seen	Postcricoid web	252
Solids worse than liquids ⟶	Endoscopy—pooling of saliva	Achalasia	253
Pain			
Otalgia			
Neck lump			
Constant			
Progressive			
Regurgitation ⟶		Pharyngeal pouch	254
Halitosis			
Liquids worse than solids ⟶	+ neurology/cranial nerve palsies ⟶	Neurological dysphagia	251
Intermittent			
Saliva worse than solids or liquids			
Variable			
With or without variable voice problems ⟶	Normal ⟶	Globus	246
Heartburn		GORD	250
Feeling of a lump in the throat			
Mucus in the throat			

A feeling of a lump in the throat

History	Examination	Diagnosis	Page no.
Constant			
Same site			
Worse with solids	Lesion seen on examination →	Carcinoma of pharynx	256
Unilateral	Palpable neck lump	Carcinoma of oesophagus	
pain			
otalgia			
neck lump			
hoarse voice			
Patient is a smoker			
Variable site			
Comes and goes			
Worse with saliva	Examination normal →	Globus	246
No true dysphagia			
Central in the neck			
Variable voice problems			
Anxiety			
Patient has a cancer phobia			
Heartburn/GORD			

A lump in the neck

All of the below may apply to children, but the majority of neck masses in children are benign and most are reactive lymph nodes. Parotid lumps in children are more frequently malignant than in adults.

History	Examination	Diagnosis	Page no.
Short history (weeks/months) ⟶	Laterally placed	Neoplastic lymphadenopathy	270
Lump is enlarging	Firm/hard	ENT primary	
Unilateral nasal obstruction	Single/multiple		
Otalgia			
Sore throat			
Patient is a smoker			
Hoarse voice			
Swallowing problems			
Weight loss ⟶	Multiple	Malignant lymphoma	270
Night sweats ⟶	Rubbery		
Anorexia	Groin/axillary nodes	Glandular fever/toxoplasmosis	269
Fever			
Foreign travel ⟶		Tuberculosis	269

Previous/recent URTI ———→	Multiple/single ———→	Reactive lymphadenopathy	269
Long history (months/years)	Single & lateral ———→	Branchial cyst	266
No associated symptoms			
	Single & midline		
	Rises on swallowing ———→	Thyroid lump	266
	Rises on tongue protrusion ———→	Thyroglossal cyst	266
	No movement or swallowing ———→	Dermoid cyst	266
		Lymph node	269
	Parotid region		
	No facial weakness ———→	Benign parotid tumour	204
	Facial weakness & pain ———→	Malignant parotid tumour	204
	Submandibular region ———→	Submandibular gland tumour	204
Changes with eating	Parotid ———→	Parotid stone/parotitis	205/207
	Submandibular ———→	Submandibular stone/sialadenitis	206/207

Mouth or tongue ulcer

History	Examination	Diagnosis	Page no.
Trauma or injury Poor fitting denture Sharp tooth Pain	Lateral tongue Buccal mucosa	→ Traumatic ulcer	188
Patient is a smoker Alcohol Betel nut chewer Progressive Pain Neck mass Otalgia	Lateral tongue Floor of mouth Tonsil Firm/hard ulcer Neck nodes	→ Malignant ulcer (SCC)	189
Normal immune function Recurrent	Multiple ulcers Tongue tip/lateral border	→ Aphthous ulcers	188
Dietary insufficiency	Angular stomatitis Skin lesions	→ Dietary/blood disorders	188

Stridor

History	Examination	Diagnosis	🔲 Page no.
Neonate			
Feeding problems	Positional ────────➤	Laryngomalacia	218
Failure to thrive		Tracheomalacia	
Abnormal cry ─────────────────────────➤		Vocal cord lesion/palsy	219
	Biphasic stridor ───➤	Subglottic stenosis	218
Child			
Preceding URTI			
Rapid onset ────────➤	Drooling	Croup	222
Malaise	Pyrexia ──────────➤	Epiglottitis	221
Voice muffled/changed	Toxic		
Short history	Inspiratory/mixed stridor ────➤	Foreign body	236
Previously well child	Expiratory wheeze		
Short-lived coughing fit			

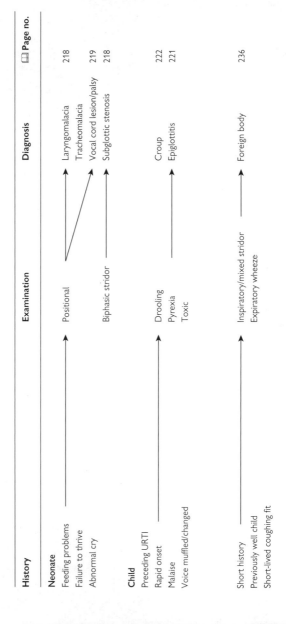

Adult

Normal voice
Recent surgery (thyroid/chest) —————————→ Inspiratory stridor —————————→ Bilateral cord palsy   231, 232

Preceding URTI
Malaise   Inspiratory stridor —————————→ Supraglottitis   221
Swallowing difficulty   Pyrexia
Sore throat   Drooling

Long-standing hoarse voice —————————→ Inspiratory stridor —————————→ Laryngeal carcinoma   224
Pain   Neck node
Patient is a smoker

Facial nerve palsy

History	Examination	Diagnosis	📖 Page no.
Recent trauma Haemotympanum	Head injury Trauma to ear canal/drum Cerebrospinal fluid (CSF) from ear/nose →	Fractured temporal bone	144
Rapid onset Other weakness	Forehead unaffected Abnormal neurological exam →	Cerebrovascular disease (CVA)	251
Rapid onset Isolated weakness	Forehead affected →	Bell's palsy	378
Otalgia	Vesicles in ear →	Ramsay Hunt	378
Gradual onset Other weakness	Abnormal neurological exam →	Multiple sclerosis (MS) Motor neurone disease	378
Gradual onset Facial pain	Parotid lump →	Parotid carcinoma	204
Hearing loss Balance disturbance	Sensorineural hearing loss ataxia →	Cerebellopontine angle (CPA) tumour	153
Ear discharge	Conductive hearing loss →	Cholesteatoma	100

Nasal obstruction

Careful examination of the nasal anatomy will reveal what is responsible for nasal obstruction. Always remember that several anatomical problems can coexist. Symptoms can vary, especially for mucosal problems, so ascertain the severity of the problem when you examine the patient's nose.

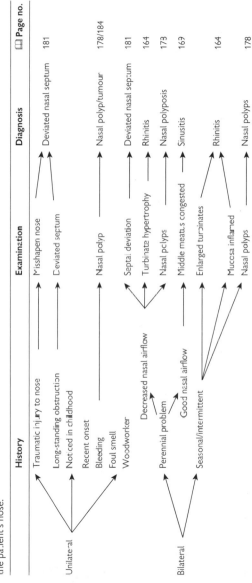

History	Examination	Diagnosis	🔲 Page no.
Traumatic injury to nose →	Misshapen nose →	Deviated nasal septum	181
Long-standing obstruction →	Deviated septum ↗		
Noticed in childhood ↗			
Recent onset			
Bleeding →	Nasal polyp →	Nasal polyp/tumour	178/184
Foul smell ↗			
Woodworker ↗	Septal deviation →	Deviated nasal septum	181
Decreased nasal airflow ↗	Turbinate hypertrophy →	Rhinitis	164
Perennial problem ↗	Nasal polyps →	Nasal polyposis	173
Good nasal airflow →	Middle meatus congested →	Sinusitis	169
Seasonal/intermittent ↗	Enlarged turbinates ↗		
	Mucosa inflamed →	Rhinitis	164
	Nasal polyps →	Nasal polyps	178

The discharging ear

The timing of the onset of discharge in relation to any pain often helps with diagnosis. Otitis externa in particular can be secondary to infection spreading from the middle ear. Microsuction, or dry mopping, is often necessary to visualize the tympanic membrane. A final diagnosis is sometimes not possible until the ear has been cleaned and the local infection has been treated. It is important to visualize the eardrum after treatment to exclude serious pathology at the level of the tympanic membrane.

History	Examination	Diagnosis	Page no.
No pain	EAC appears normal and the tympanic membrane (TM) appears to have attic retraction/keratin	Cholesteatoma	100
	EAC appears normal and the TM is perforated or has grommets	CSOM/infected grommet	98
Pain before discharge	Normal EAC with a bulging TM	Acute otitis media	94
	Granulations in floor of EAC with a normal TM	Necrotizing otitis externa	84
Pain after discharge	Narrow oedematous EAC when the TM is normal or not seen	Otitis externa	82

Dizziness and vertigo

The most important aspect here is the patient's history. Take great care to elicit the character of the dizziness and its timecourse to establish if this is dizziness or true vertigo.

	History	Examination	Diagnosis	📖 Page no.
True vertigo	Lasts for **seconds**	Dix-Hallpike test +ve	BPPV	135
	Positional			
	Lasts for **hours**	Pure tone audiometry fluctuating (PTA) sensorineural loss (sometimes low tone affected)	Ménière's	138
	Aural fullness			
	Fluctuating hearing loss			
	Recurrent episodes			
	Lasts for **days**	FTA normal	Vestibular neuronitis	134
	Single severe attack	Unterberger's test +ve	Vascular causes	142
	Unwell for 1 week			
Disequilibrium	Constant	PTA normal	Multifactorial causes	
	Elderly patient	Vestibular function tests normal		
	Intermittent	PTA normal	Decompensation	134
	Previous severe attack of vertigo			

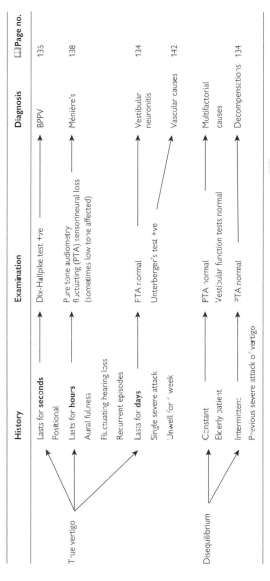

Otalgia (earache)

Patients who present with otalgia can present a challenging problem. A careful history can help distinguish many conditions. Beware the red reflex—a reflex dilatation of the blood vessels on the handle of the malleus caused by the otoscope speculum touching the bony ear canal. This is often misdiagnosed as early acute otitis media, and the true cause of otalgia is missed. Always consider if the otalgia is referred pain.

History		Examination (using an otoscope)	Diagnosis	📖 Page no.
Severe pain Child/preceding upper respiratory tract infection (URTI) Very painful	→	Erythema—a bulging drum A high temperature Distressed patient	Acute otitis media	94
Severe pain Preceding itch Longstanding Surfer/swimmer	Not diabetic →	Narrow EAC Mucopus	Otitis externa	82
Severe pain Elderly	Diabetic →	EAC floor granulated Patient unwell Cranial nerve palsies	Necrotizing otitis externa	84
Intermittent severe pain At night time Known glue ear	→	Middle ear effusion	Glue ear	97
Severe pain Anterior to tragus Worse with eating	→	Normal TM Tender over temporomandibular joint (TMJ) Malaligned bite	TMJ dysfunction	
Moderate/severe	→	Normal TM	Referred pain	198

Hearing loss

A diagnosis of hearing loss in children and adults depends on combining the information from the patient's history, the examination and any special investigations. An audiogram, or a tympanogram with tuning fork tests will help to distinguish conductive from sensorineural hearing loss and will determine if the problem is bilateral or affects only one ear. Sudden hearing loss is an emergency.

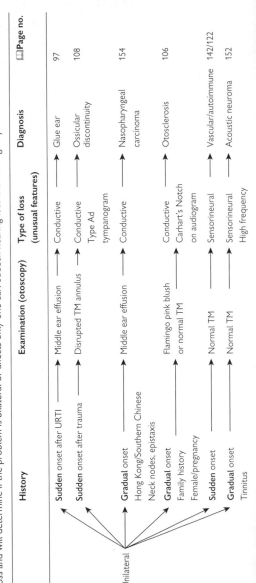

History	Examination (otoscopy)	Type of loss (unusual features)	Diagnosis	📖 Page no.
Sudden onset after URTI	Middle ear effusion	Conductive	Glue ear	97
Sudden onset after trauma	Disrupted TM annulus	Conductive Type Ad tympanogram	Ossicular discontinuity	108
Gradual onset Hong Kong/Southern Chinese Neck nodes, epistaxis	Middle ear effusion	Conductive	Nasopharyngeal carcinoma	154
Gradual onset Family history Female/pregnancy	Flamingo pink blush or normal TM	Conductive Carhart's Notch on audiogram	Otosclerosis	106
Sudden onset	Normal TM	Sensorineural	Vascular/autoimmune	142/122
Gradual onset Tinnitus	Normal TM	Sensorineural High frequency	Acoustic neuroma	152

Unilateral

Bilateral

Gradual onset
Child → Middle ear effusion → Conductive
Type B tympanogram → Glue ear ... 97

Sudden onset → Normal TM → Sensorineural → Autoimmune ... 122

Gradual onset
Elderly → Normal TM → Sensorineural → Presbyacusis ... 116

Gradual onset
Noise exposure → Normal TM → Sensorineural
Audiogram notch
at 4KHz → Noise-induced
hearing loss (NIHL) ... 118

Tinnitus

It is important to distinguish between objective tinnitus (which the examiner can hear) and subjective tinnitus (which only the patient can hear). The character of the tinnitus is also important. A thorough otoneurological examination—of the ears, cranial nerves, and central nervous system—is essential. Auscultate the ear, eye, and carotids. Remember that tinnitus can be caused by medication or other drugs.

Character of tinnitus	Laterality	Examination	Diagnosis	📖 Page no.
Pulsatile	Unilateral	Abnormal TM or middle ear mass	Glomus tumour	
		Objective tinnitus Normal PTA	Arteriovenous malformation	142
	Bilateral	Normal TM	Carotid stenosis	
		Subjective tinnitus Normal PTA	Psychogenic (beware using this label too frequently)	
Non-pulsatile → Humming	Unilateral	Normal TM	Acoustic neuroma	152
		High-frequency asymmetric sensorineural hearing loss (SNHL)		
	Bilateral	Wax impaction	Foreign body	362
		Normal TM	Presbyacusis	116
		High-frequency symmetric loss		
Clicking	Bilateral	SNHL with 4kHz notch	NIHL	118
		Normal examination		
	Unilateral	Objective tinnitus	Tensor tympani contraction	

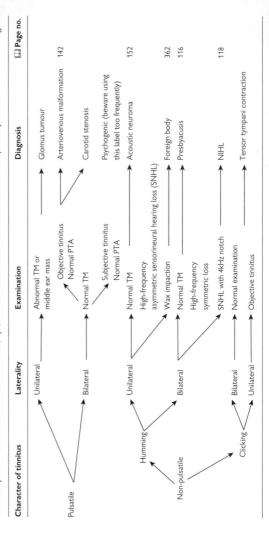

Facial pain

Patients with this problem may present to a variety of specialties for an opinion, e.g. ENT, neurology, or maxillofacial surgery. It is important to have a broad mind to avoid a misdiagnosis. Never be afraid to ask for another specialist's opinion.

History	Examination	Diagnosis	📖 Page no.
Severe acute pain Pain periorbital/cheeks Provoked by URTI Nasal obstruction Temperature	→ Pus/polyps in middle meatus →	Acute sinusitis	169
Chronic fullness Worse bending over Nasal obstruction	→ Middle meatus occluded/narrowed →	Chronic sinusitis	172
Severe pain Localized to specific site No nasal obstruction No rhinitic symptoms	→ Normal nasal examination Normal nasendoscopy →	Atypical facial pain	
Intermittent pain Worse on eating Radiates to ear	→ Normal nasal examination Normal nasendoscopy Tenderness over TMJ →	TMJ dysfunction	

Investigations in ENT

Pure tone audiometry (PTA)

This is the most common method used for assessing hearing. The examination will ideally take place in a soundproof booth. To avoid cheating, the patient should not be able to see the audiometer controls.

The examiner and the patient are in contact via a microphone and a headset. The patient wears headphones and is given a hand-held button to press when they hear a sound during the test. The better hearing ear is tested first.

The test begins using air-conducted sounds. Initially, sound is played through the headphones at a level above the hearing threshold. The sound is decreased in 10dB increments until it is no longer heard. The sound intensity is then increased in 5dB increments until a 50% response rate is obtained.

- The different frequencies (notes) by convention are tested in the following order: 1kHz, 2kHz, 4kHz, 8kHz, 500Hz, 250Hz, and then 1kHz again.
- The re-test at 1kHz should be within 10dB of the initial result.
- The test–retest error is approximately 5dB.

The test is then repeated using bone conduction. The bone conductor is tightly applied to the mastoid area where the skin is tethered to the bone more securely and better contact is obtained.

Masking

Like tuning fork testing, there is a potential source of error in the pure tone audiogram. This is because sound can be perceived in the non-test ear if it is conducted through bone or through the air.

Masking is when white noise is applied to the non-test ear via air conduction in order to block it out and remove it from the test. This ensures it cannot interfere with the results from the test ear.

Consider masking when:
- the air conduction thresholds of both ears show a difference of >40dB
- testing air conduction, the unmasked bone thresholds are 40dB better than the worst air conduction
- testing bone conduction, the difference between the unmasked bone is better than the worst air conduction by 10dB or more.

These scenarios enable the true hearing thresholds of both ears to be measured, and avoids picking up a false-positive result from an ear that has no hearing at all!

The results are recorded on a chart. (◻ See Fig. 4.1.)

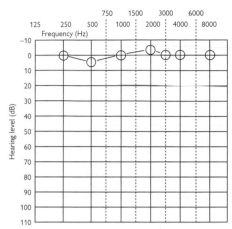

Fig. 4.1 Normal hearing (right ear). Reproduced from *Diseases of the Ear* (Harold Ludman and Tony Wright), with permission of Edward Arnold (Publishers) Ltd © 1997 Arnold.

Tympanometry

Tympanometry is a way of measuring the pressure in the middle ear. It was developed and popularized by Jerger as a way of establishing the cause of conductive deafness. He classified the different patterns described opposite.

Method

- The EAC is checked with an otoscope to ensure that there is no infection or debris blocking the EAC.
- The test probe is placed in the external auditory meatus to give a tight seal to the external ear canal (EAC). This seal is facilitated by using soft tip ends. The probe varies the pressure in the EAC whilst firing a 225Hz sound signal at the tympanic membrane (TM) or ear drum.
- The probe then measures the amount of sound reflected from the TM and calculates how much of the sound energy is admitted. Most sound is admitted when the pressure in the EAC matches that of the middle ear space. Thus the instrument measures the compliance of the tympanic membrane.
- By calculating the amount of air needed to change the EAC pressure, the machine also calculates an approximate EAC volume.
- The test is fast, comfortable and can be performed on children of any age.

Uses

- Determining the cause of a conductive hearing loss
- Screening for the presence of glue ear
- Checking the patency of a grommet
- Checking for a microscopic perforation of the tympanic membrane
- Assessing Eustachian tube function

Problems

- User-dependent
- Cannot be used with extensive infection or debris blocking the EAC
- Occasionally, air leakage from the EAC can give a false-positive result for a Type B tympanogram

Interpretation of results

- Does the trace have a definite peak?
- At which EAC pressure does the peak occur?
- Is the ear canal volume greater than 1cm^3?

Classification of results (Fig. 4.2)

Type A—Normal waveform with definite peak showing maximum admittance at atmospheric pressure (0 on Fig. 4.2). Variations occur:
- **As**—where peak is at 0 but height of peak is diminished, e.g. stiff ossicular chain
- **Ad**— where peak is abnormally high in ossicular chain dislocation

Type B—Trace is a flat line. Can be due to a middle ear effusion where the fluid in the middle ear space is incompressible and admittance does not change with varying pressure changes in the EAC. Calculated EAC canal volume is normal. When there is a flat trace and EAC volume is high ($>1cm^3$) this usually indicates a tympanic membrane perforation or the presence of a patent grommet.

Type C—Peak occurs at a negative pressure. Due to low middle ear pressure from Eustachian tube dysfunction.
- **C1**—peak lies between 0 and −200kPa
- **C2**—peak lies between −200 and −400kPa

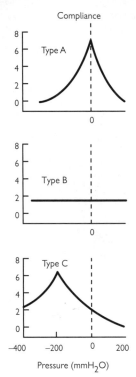

Fig. 4.2 Types of tympanogram.

Otoacoustic emissions (OAEs)

The cochlea has been postulated to generate sound. This was first recorded and documented by Kemp in the 1970s. The sound is believed to originate from the outer hair cells in the cochlea. These cells actively contract to modify the travelling wave produced by sound in the cochlea to make the wave have a sharp well-defined peak which is frequency-specific. During this active process some of the sound vibration produced by the outer hair cells escapes through the middle ear and can be recorded in the external auditory canal. The sounds can either be produced spontaneously or induced from the application of sounds to the outer ear. Absence of recordable OAEs has been shown to correlate with pathology of the ear

Different types of OAEs are recognized:

- *Spontaneously evoked (SOAEs)*—Recordings of cochlea sounds without stimulation
- *Transient evoked (TEOAEs)*—Cochlea sounds recorded in response to clicks or tone bursts applied to the EAC
- *Distortion product (DPOAEs)*—Cochlea sounds produced in response to two distinct tones of different frequencies applied to the ear at the same time
- *Single frequency (SFOAEs)*—Cochlea sounds produced in response to a single continuous tone

Technique
- The EAC is checked for occlusion.
- A probe is applied to the EAC using an age-specific flexible soft tip.
- Sound is applied to the ear via the probe and simultaneous recordings of the sounds emitted from the ear are made. A computer analyses these recordings.

Uses
- Universal newborn hearing screening
- Objective assessment of hearing in incapacitated subjects
- Objective measure in assessing non-organic hearing loss

Problems
- User-dependent
- Occluded EAC due to infection
- Middle ear pathology, e.g. glue ear inhibits recording of OAEs, but can be used with grommets
- False-negative if hearing problem is due to neurological involvement and cochlea function is normal

Interpretation of results

OAEs can only be used to assess the function of the cochlea. There is a strong correlation between the presence of OAEs and a normal functioning cochlea. Fortunately, most cochlea disease causes equal damage and loss of inner and outer hair cells. This enables the function of the outer hair cells, which produce the noise, to be used as a marker of ear function. The commonest types of OAEs used clinically are the

TEOAEs and the DPOAEs. They have different uses and are often complimentary:

- **TEOAEs** are fast, sensitive to losses of up to 15–20dB, but become less sensitive at frequencies greater than 4KHz. (More commonly used in neonatal screening).
- **DPOAEs** are less sensitive, but still are sensitive to losses in the range 25 to 30dB; their sensitivity does not drop off at higher frequencies.

Both provide some frequency-specific information. Each OAE is produced from a particular area of the cochlea. This depends on the stimulus. TEOAEs use clicks which have a wide range of frequencies. Responses will be recorded but any damaged area of the cochlea will not produce a response. DPOAEs use two different frequencies for stimulus and the response will be a function of the two frequencies. Variation of the frequencies can give data on different regions of the cochlea.

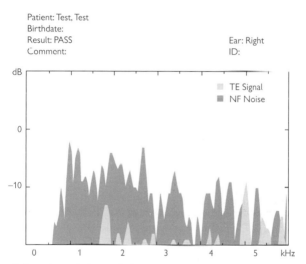

Patient: Test, Test
Birthdate:
Result: PASS
Comment:
Ear: Right
ID:

Right: 24-Apr-07: Stab:100% : TE Screen, 70% at 3/4 freq. for pass: 07D23T00.TE

Frq (kHz)	Repro (%)	TE (dB)	NF (dB)	TE-NF (dB)	Result
1.0	97	4.5	−9.6	14.1	−
1.5	96	1.0	−10.0	11.0	Pass
2.0	83	5.3	−4.5	9.8	Pass
3.0	88	4.5	−6.1	10.6	Pass
4.0	73	2.7	−4.8	7.5	Pass
1.2–3.5	87	8.8	−1.6	10.4	−

Fig. 4.3 Transient evoked OAE (TEOAE). Reproduced with permission from Warner et al., *Otolaryngology and Head and Neck Surgery*, 2009 © Oxford University Press.

Auditory brainstem response (ABR)

This test refers to the recording of electrical activity along the auditory pathway in response to a sound stimulus. The characteristic waveform produced is believed to represent the sequential firing of neurons from the VIIIth nerve initially to the brainstem.

Technique

- Assess ear for the presence of an effusion. Use otoscopy and tympanometry. Grommets are required if it is present.
- For adults, carry out the test in a soundproof room.
- Sedate young children, e.g. with trimeprazine 4mg/kg followed by 2mg/kg 1 hour later if the child is still active.
- General anaesthesia can be used, especially if grommets need to be inserted.
- Deliver sound stimulus (provided by repetitive clicks) via headphones. Masking can be required if evoked thresholds differ by more than 50dB between the ears.
- Position electrodes:
  - active electrode—vertex of the scalp.
  - reference electrode—ipsilateral ear lobe
  - earth electrode—forehead
- Record waveform in response to sound stimulus.
- Repeat test with decreasing sound stimulus intensity until characteristic waveform is not seen. This is the likely audiological hearing threshold.
- Repeat the test for the other ear.

Problems

- User-dependent—relies on waveform interpretation.
- Cannot be used with middle ear effusions.

Uses

- Neonatal universal hearing screening
- Objective assessment of hearing thresholds
- Identification of retrocochlear pathology
- Intraoperative monitoring

Interpretation of results

The classical waveform is produced as seen in Fig. 4.4.
- Wave I: Action potential of auditory nerve
- Wave II: Proximal region of auditory nerve
- Wave III: Cochlear nucleus
- Wave IV: Superior olive
- Wave V: Lateral lemniscus
- Wave VI: Inferior colliculus
- Wave VII: Inferior colliculus

SN10: slow negative wave, associated with Wave V, with a 10ms latency (midbrain origin)

Features suggesting retrocochlear pathology, e.g. acoustic neuroma

- Delay in the development of Wave V.
- Failure to record a waveform.
- Sensitivity 90% and specificity 80% (MRI essential)

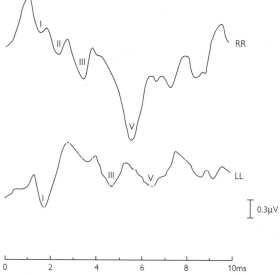

Fig. 4.4 Normal ABR (above) compared to abnormal ABR. Reproduced from *Diseases of the Ear* (Harold Ludman and Tony Wright), with permission of Edward Arnold (Publishers) Ltd © 1997 Arnold.

ENG and calorics

These are balance tests.

Electronystagmography (ENG) measures the chorioretinal electrical potential difference. Electrodes placed near the eyes can pick up electrical changes caused by eye movements. ENG allows testing of the vestibulo-ocular reflex (VOR). The VOR allows clear vision during head movements by producing compensatory eye movements.

The ENG test is usually performed in a dimly lit room with a light bar to provide visual calibration. The patient sits on the examination couch.

Uses of ENG

ENG enables an assessment of the following:
- Disorders in squamous cell carcinoma (SCC) and otolith organs
- Integrity of brainstem–cerebellar pathways
- Integrity of central vestibulo-ocular pathways

Subtests

If a patient needs more detailed investigations, they may be sent for more tests which may include:
- Oculomotor control test:
  - saccades
  - tracking/smooth pursuit
  - optokinetic test
  - gaze test
- Positional testing:
  - headshake
  - Dix–Hallpike test
- Caloric tests:
  - warm and cold irrigations
  - ice calorics
  - fixation tests

Calorics

This test involves warm or cold water being squirted into the ear. This stimulates the inner ear balance mechanisms and will make the patient dizzy. The degree of dizziness can be measured by observing the nystagmus that is produced. This test is performed on both sides and any difference is an indication of pathology in the balance system. It is used to confirm an inner ear cause of a balance problem.

Procedure
- Irrigate with warm water at 44°C and cool the EAC at 30°C for 30 seconds with 200ml of fluid. (Alternatively, use warm air at 50°C and cool at 24°C for 60 seconds at 9L/min flow rate.) The temperature difference stimulates eddy currents in the lateral SCC.
- Nystagmus induced according to COWS (Cold Opposite Warm the Same)
- Compare responses according to the formula below.

Unilateral Weakness 25% significance

$$\frac{(RC+RW) - (LC+LW)}{RC+LC+RW+LW} \times 100 = \text{Unilateral Weakness}$$

Directional Preponderance 25–30% significance

$$\frac{(RC+LW) - (LC+RW)}{\textbf{RC+LC+RW+LW}} \times 100 = \text{Directional Preponderance}$$

Children's hearing assessment

Assessing the hearing of babies and children can be difficult, because most hearing tests involve the active co-operation of the participant. To get round this problem, a number of tests have been specially designed for children; and different tests are used at different ages.

Universal neonatal screening

The incidence of children born with sensorineural hearing loss is estimated as between 1 and 3 per 1000 live births.

Early detection is necessary to avoid:
- Social problems
- Psychological problems

Begin rehabilitation as early as possible.
   Techniques used are:
- Otoacoustic emissions (📖 see 'Otoacoustic emissions', p. 60)
- ABR (📖 see 'Auditory brainstem response', p. 62)

Distraction testing

This test is usually done by health visitors, as part of the routine health screening of infants at nine months of age. Two testers are required for this examination. The child sits on the parent's or carer's lap, and one of the examiners sits in front of the child to occupy its attention. The other tester stands behind the child and uses sounds of particular frequency and volume to stimulate the child to turn its head. Turning is a positive response.

Visual reinforcement audiometry

This test is similar to distraction testing, but it uses speakers or headphones to deliver the unilateral sound. If the child turns round correctly then a light or a toy turns on to reward their turning.

Conditioned response audiometry

The child is conditioned to perform a task in response to a sound; for example, putting a toy man into a toy boat.

McCormick toy testing

This test uses 12 paired toys or objects with similar sounding names, e.g. a cup and a duck. The child points to or picks up the correct toy. The intensity of the sound of the command can be changed. The child's hearing threshold is determined by an 80% response.

Pure tone audiogram

This test can sometimes be performed by children as young as three years old. PTA using bone conduction can be uncomfortable for younger children (📖 see 'Pure tone audiogram', p. 54).

Tympanometry

This test measures pressure in the middle ear and is useful and accurate in detecting glue ear.

CT scan

Computed tomography (CT) provides excellent information for defining differences between bony and soft tissue. In ENT it is used for looking for problems affecting the temporal bone and the inner ear.

The patient lies supine on the scanner bed. The scan uses X-rays applied in a circumferential manner to acquire information. Information is produced in the form of pixel cubes. These can be joined to produce images in multiple planes. There is a significant radiation dose with this technique.

Uses

- Evaluation of bony anatomy for endoscopic sinus surgery
- Evaluation of mandibular involvement in floor of mouth tumours
- Assessment of middle ear in suspected mastoiditis
- Evaluation of traumatic head injury and temporal bone fracture

MRI scan

This technique provides excellent soft tissue definition with no radiation risk. In ENT it is used for looking at the nerves to and from the inner ear.

The patient is placed lying down, inside a circular magnet. The magnetic field aligns all the hydrogen atoms, mainly body water. An electromagnetic pulse is directed towards the patient, which knocks the hydrogen atoms out of alignment. Once the pulse wave has subsided the hydrogen atoms spring back into alignment. This process causes energy to be released, which is detected by the scanner.

The timing of recording, and the information collected can be analysed separately to give different information. Software algorithms produce the 3D image information. Contrast can enhance the information.

Common protocols

- T1 weighted scans
- T2 weighted scans
- STIR sequence (short tau inversion recovery) produces fat-suppressed images
- Magnetic resonance angiography (MRA) gives angiographic information from the scan sequence

Uses

- Identifying acoustic neuroma—MRI is the gold standard
- Checking the spread of a tumour
- Assessing the involvement of vascular structures in head and neck malignancy
- Assessing the intracranial spread of sinonasal tumours

Allergy testing

Skin prick testing

This test enables you to detect if a patient is allergic to various substances. It has an instant result, allowing you to see the allergic response. Skin prick testing (SPT) is used extensively in patients with rhinitis, to guide therapy, and to aid advice on which allergens to avoid.

Procedure

- The patient is asked to refrain from taking antihistamines for 48 hours prior to testing.
- Before starting this test, it is important to ensure that resuscitation facilities are nearby, with adrenaline.
- The procedure for testing should be explained to the patient. The test solutions are then placed on the patient's forearm. These include a positive control substance (histamine) and a negative control substance (excipient solution—the chemical that the allergens are diluted into). A small amount of solution is inoculated intradermally by using a lancet pricked into the patient's skin (puncture test).
- A positive response, shown as a wheal >2 mm, is measured after 30 minutes. The wheal lasts about an hour.

Common antigens tested

- House dust
- House dust mite
- Tree mix
- Dog dander
- Cat dander
- Moulds
- Grass

Advantages

Cheap, easy to perform, results in 30 minutes. More specific and sensitive than RAST tests.

Disadvantages

Slightly uncomfortable, children may not co-operate can be unreliable in the elderly and in <2 year olds

RAST tests

RAST stands for radioallergosorbent testing. This is a blood test which detects circulating IgE to specific antigens. It is more expensive than SPTs. It takes about 7 days to obtain a result.

Uses

- Unco-operative patient who cannot undergo SPTs
- Unable to stop antihistamines
- Severe eczema so that skin tests cannot be performed
- Risk of anaphylactic shock in very sensitive patients
- Rare allergen suspected

Results

Levels of detectable IgE are classified in Table 4.1.

Table 4.1 Sensitivity of RAST

Level	Amount (kU/L)	Result
0	<0.35	Negative result
1	0.35–0.69	
2	0.7–3.4	
3	3.5–17.4	
4	17.5–49.9	
5	50–99	
6	>100	Very high sensitivity

The external ear

Structure and function of the external ear

A working knowledge of the anatomy of the ear helps in documentation, correspondence, and in describing sites of lesions and trauma over the telephone. The main anatomical points are shown in Figs 5.1 and 5.2.

The external part of the ear consists of two parts:
• The pinna
• The external auditory canal (EAC).

The pinna collects sound waves and directs them into the external auditory canal. Its shape aids localization of sound direction and amplification.

The EAC transmits sound waves to the eardrum or tympanic membrane.
The EAC has two parts:
• An outer cartilaginous part
• An inner bony part.

In adults, the cartilaginous canal slopes forward and downward.
In neonates and infants, the canal slopes forward.
The outer canal contains hairs and ceruminous glands that produce wax.

(a)

(b)

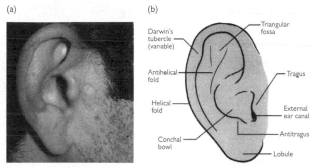

Darwin's tubercle (variable)

Triangular fossa

Antihelical fold

Tragus

Helical fold

External ear canal

Antitragus

Conchal bowl

Lobule

Fig. 5.1 The pinna.

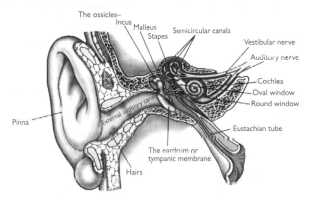

The ossicles—

Incus

Malleus

Stapes

Semicircular canals

Vestibular nerve

Auditory nerve

Cochlea

Oval window

Round window

External auditory canal

Eustachian tube

Pinna

The eardrum or tympanic membrane

Hairs

Fig. 5.2 Diagram of the EAC.

Congenital abnormalities

Minor abnormalities of the ear are common, but often they do not come to medical attention.

Malformed pinna

The pinna develops from the six hillocks of His. Maldevelopment or failure to fuse can produce obvious abnormalities of the ear. Malformed pinnae are described as 'microtia' or 'anotia'. They may or may not be associated with middle or inner ear abnormalities. The various classifications are shown in Fig. 5.3.

Investigations

- Documentation of the defect
- EAC examination
- Hearing assessment
- CT scan to assess middle ear/ossicles/cochlea anatomy may also be required

Treatment

Where there are minor anatomical abnormalities, no treatment is given; hearing support is given as required.

Where there is a major deformity or anotia, removal of the pinna may be considered. Reconstruction can be facilitated using titanium osseo-integrated implants. These are surgically inserted into the bone and can be used to attach an artificial pinna or a bone-anchored hearing aid (BAHA).

Skin tags

Skin tags are often detected at a neonatal baby check. They are often incidental findings and investigations should simply involve checking for normal EAC and screening hearing tests.

Preauricular sinus

This is a small dimple anterior to the tragus, which may be the external opening of a network of channels under the skin (Fig. 5.4). It is usually detected at a baby check and is caused by the incomplete fusion of the hillocks of His. Patients who present late may have a discharge from the punctum. Occasionally, repeated infections may require drainage.

Treatment

Where there is simple discharge—treat with oral antibiotics such as co-amoxiclav (e.g. Augmentin). Antibiotics may be given and surgical removal may be necessary in patients with repeated infections.

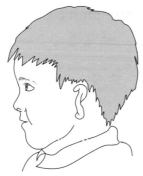

Fig. 5.3 Diagram of microtia grade III. Grading of microtia—I: normal ear; II: all pinna elements present but malformed; III: rudimentary bar only; IV: anotia.

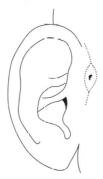

Fig. 5.4 Diagram of preauricular sinus.

Infection of the pinna

This presents as a painful, hot, red ear.

Assessment

- Identify the cause of the infection. Is this a spreading infection from the EAC or is it a primary infection of the pinna?
- Identify whether it is an infection of the skin or does it also involve cartilage? If the cartilage is infected there is severe tenderness on touching the pinna.
- Take a history and exclude trauma or an insect bite. Remember non-accidental injury in children. Diabetic or immunocompromised patients may have severe cellulitis of the pinna.

Treatment

- Where there is a localized infection—remove any cause such as piercing or an insect's sting. Give oral antibiotics such as co-amoxiclav 625mg tds for 1 week PO.
- Where there is cellulitis of the pinna—remove the cause and treat with IV antibiotics such as cefuroxime 1.5g tds and metronidazole 500mg tds IV until the cellulitis resolves; continue for at least 24 hours followed by oral antibiotics for 1 week in total.
- Where there is perichondritis—remove the cause or treat otitis externa if present. Treat with IV antibiotics such as cefuroxime 1.5g tds and metronidazole 500mg tds IV until the cellulitis resolves; continue for at least 24 hours followed by oral antibiotics for 1 week in total.

Piercings

The current fashion trend dictates that piercings are often multiple and not always in the lobule of the ear. Lobule piercings have less likelihood of becoming infected as there is no cartilage in the lobule.

Other piercings transfix the cartilage framework of the pinna. This can lead to infection and cellulitis of the pinna.

Trauma to the pinna

Assess the patient, bearing in mind that a blow to the ear is a head injury. Discover the force and mechanism of the injury. The site of the injury should be carefully documented with the help of a diagram or a photograph.

Any blunt trauma to the ear may cause a hearing loss or a traumatic perforation of the eardrum. Always examine the EAC and drum and perform a simple bedside hearing assessment as follows:

- Examine the pinna and note the findings
- Examine the EAC
- Examine the tympanic membrane
- Perform tuning fork tests
- Perform free field testing of hearing
- Check patient's tetanus status

Lacerations of the skin

These are simply repaired, using non-absorbable sutures such as 5.0 Prolene. Apply local anaesthetic to the area, clean the wound, and use interrupted sutures. Pay careful attention to everting the edges and ensuring good opposition of the skin edges. Check the patient's tetanus status.

Lacerations involving the cartilage

Clean wounds can be simply sutured in layers to include the cartilage. The cartilage is very painful to suture and a general anaesthetic should be considered.

Dirty wounds may need surgical debridement under general anaesthetic (GA) before closure. All wounds require antibiotic cover, such as co-amoxiclav 625mg tds PO.

Haematoma of the pinna

This is a collection of blood between the perichondrium and the cartilage which can lead to pressure necrosis of the cartilage. Subsequent deformity, infection, and fibrosis with cartilage loss, leads to the typical 'cauliflower ear' seen in rugby players.

Aspiration of the haematoma is difficult due to the thickness of the clot. It is better to incise the haematoma and suture, using bolsters to prevent reaccumulation. ▢ See Fig. 5.5.

Treatment:

- Local anaesthetic or GA
- Incision over haematoma
- Primary closure
- Dental roll bolsters tied in place
- Removal of dressing after 5 days
- Oral antibiotics, e.g. co-amoxiclav 625 mg tds PO for 1 week.

(a) (b)

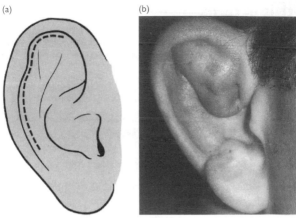

Fig. 5.5 Haematoma in the pinna.

Otitis externa

This common condition forms a large percentage of both the emergency and the routine workload of an ENT department. Its presentation is varied and it produces a spectrum of disorders which are classified below.

Risk factors
- Swimmers and surfers
- Daily hairwashers
- Diabetics
- Psoriasis sufferers
- People with an abnormal migration of keratin

Assessment
- Is the pinna normal? If there is cellulitis, admission may be needed—severe otitis externa OE
- What is the appearance of the EAC after cleaning under microscope?
- Is the EAC normal diameter?—mild OE
- Is the EAC narrow but the tympanic membrane is still visible?—moderate OE
- Is the EAC narrow but the TM is not visible due to oedema?—severe OE
- Is there a furuncle in the EAC?
- Are there granulations in the floor of the EAC?—this may be necrotizing OE (□ see 'Necrotizing otitis externa', p. 84)
- What is the patient's facial nerve function?—test

Treatment
All patients should keep their ears water-free during treatment.

Mild OE
Presentation: scaly skin on appearance with some erythema.
- Use either 0.5% hydrocortisone cream prn to be applied to the EAC
- Or Betnovate® scalp lotion
- Or Earcalm® Spray (contains acetic acid). Lowering the pH changes the flora of the EAC
- Regular aural toilet and avoid water entering the ears during bathing and no swimming

Moderate OE
Presentation: painful, discharging, smelly ears. Narrowed EAC with creamy, cheese-like discharge.
- Microsuction clearance
- Swab for microscopy if there has been previous antibiotic treatment
- Otowick if the EAC very narrow
- Hygroscopic drops, e.g. aluminium acetate
- Change wick in 48 hours
- Swab if no improvement. Consider combination therapy with antibiotic steroid drops depending on swab result and response to treatment

Severe OE

Presentation: complete occlusion of the EAC or spreading pinna cellulitis

- Microsuction clearance
- Treat as moderate OE
- If there is severe pain, it may be furunculosis. Lance boil with fine end of sucker. Add flucloxacillin 500mg qds PO to regime
- If there is cellulitis, admission for IV antibiotics may be needed
- Exclude any disease of the tympanic membrane during treatment, e.g. perforation or cholesteatoma. This will become easier as the swelling settles and the TM becomes visible.

Beware of allergy

Patients not responding to the appropriate therapy may be allergic to the constituents of the drops. Patch testing by a local dermatologist may help to elucidate this problem. Betnovate® scalp lotion can be useful as it has none of the excipients that can cause allergy difficulties.

Necrotizing otitis externa

This is an uncommon severe ear infection where the infection spreads beyond the ear canal and into the surrounding tissues and bone of the skull base. It was formerly known as 'malignant otitis externa', due to the mortality associated with the condition. It is usually seen in diabetic or immunocompromised patients. If you see a diabetic patient with otitis externa, consider this condition.

Signs and symptoms

- *Pseudomonas* spp. are commonly found on culture
- Otalgia out of proportion to the clinical appearance of the EAC
- Granulation tissue in the floor of the EAC at the junction of the bony and cartilaginous parts of the canal
- Microvascular disease predisposes to an osteomyelitis which spreads across the skull base. Cranial nerves VII and IX–XII may be affected if the infection reaches the petrous apex. The opposite side of the skull base can also be affected.

Management

- Admit patient for assessment
- Take a full history
- Make a thorough ENT examination
- Check cranial nerves
- Perform aural toilet
- Consider a biopsy of the ear canal under GA/ local anaesthetic (LA)
- Do a CT scan to examine the appearance of the skull base and to stage the extent of the disease.
- Give ciprofloxacin drops, 2 drops bd
- Give oral ciprofloxacin 500mg bd PO
- Involve the infectious disease team for expert help
- Continue with drug therapy for 6–12 weeks
- Perform a surgical debridement only if the patient does not respond to medical treatment or if there is skull base extension. Surgical interventions are rare due to high mortality

Beware malignancy

If things fail to settle or if the condition progresses, don't forget there may be a possible malignant cause. An initial negative biopsy may be wrong. Consider further deep biopsy or cortical mastoidectomy for histology.

Malignancy of the pinna

The pinna is a common site for malignant skin lesions to develop.
Cancers are most commonly basal cell carcinomas (BCC), squamous cell carcinomas (SCC), and malignant melanomas.

Risk factors
- Sun exposure
- Previous skin cancers
- Chemical exposure
- Xeroderma pigmentosum

Investigations and treatment

It is sometimes possible to make a diagnosis on clinical examination. Excision biopsy with histological analysis of the specimen is the preferred treatment. Further wider excision with or without grafting can be performed.

Special reconstructions of the pinna

The unique appearance and structure of the pinna leads to several novel methods of reconstruction following tumour removal. These aim to preserve the structure of the pinna and its cosmetic appearance without compromising curative removal (Fig. 5.6).

If there is gross cartilage involvement, it may be necessary to remove the pinna entirely.

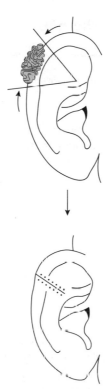

Fig. 5.6 Diagram of wedge resection.

Malignancy of the EAC

This is a rare condition, but it forms an important differential diagnosis in dealing with infections or masses in the ear. When seen, it usually affects the elderly.

SCC is the commonest type of malignancy.

Signs and symptoms
- A growth in the EAC
- Otitis externa
- Facial nerve palsy
- Other cranial nerve palsies such as IX–XII
- Lymph node metastases

Management
- Treat any infection
- Biopsy the lesion
- CT scan to stage the lesion
- MRI scan to assess intracranial spread

Treatment options
- Palliative
- Curative:
  - *radiotherapy*—thought to be inadequate for primary curative treatment. Used as an adjunct in stage T3/T4 disease
  - *surgery*—this involves lateral temporal bone resection. Superficial parotidectomy and neck dissection may also form part of the surgical excision.

Prognosis
- The outlook for these patients depends on disease stage, histology. and treatment.
- Early stage tumours: 80–100% 5-year survival
- Advanced lesions: 0–40% 2-year survival

Pittsburgh staging for external ear canal tumours
T1—Tumour limited to the EAC without bony erosion or evidence of soft tissue involvement

T2—Tumour with limited EAC bone erosion (not full thickness) with <0.5cm soft tissue involvement

T3—Tumour eroding the bony EAC with <0.5cm soft tissue involvement or tumour involving the middle ear, mastoid, or both

T4—Tumour eroding the cochlea, petrous apex, medial wall of the middle ear, carotid canal, or jugular foramen of dura; or with extensive soft tissue involvement (>0.5cm), such as involvement of the temporo-mandibular joint or stylomastoid foramen; or with evidence of facial paresis

The middle ear

Structure and function of the middle ear

The function of the middle ear is to transduce sound waves, amplify them, and pass them to the cochlea. There is also an intrinsic mechanism to protect the ear from loud noise.

The middle ear is made up of the following structures:
- The tympanic membrane
- The ossicular chain
- Nerves of the middle ear
- Muscles of the middle ear
- Mastoid air cell system
- Eustachian tube

Tympanic membrane

The TM is divided into the pars flaccida and the pars tensa by the anterior and posterior malleolar folds. Although the entire drum is composed of three layers, the two pars differ in their strength. The pars tensa has collagen fibres arranged radially, while the pars flaccida has randomly arranged collagen and a high elastin content. The squamous epithelium of the outer layer grows from central drum germinal centres. It then migrates radially and out along the EAC to be shed at the EAM.

The ossicular chain

The malleus, incus, and stapes conduct and amplify sound. The difference in contact area between the drum and the malleus compared to the contact area between the stapes and the oval window leads to an amplification. When this is added to the mechanical advantage of the articulated ossicular chain, the total amplification is in the order of 22 times.

Nerves of the middle ear

The facial nerve has an intricate course. The chorda tympani is a branch of the facial nerve. The tympanic plexus supplies secretomotor fibres to the parotid.

Muscles of the middle ear

The stapedius contracts and dampens the movement of stapes. The tensor tympani contracts and stabilizes the movement of the malleus. Both these mechanisms protect the ear from loud noise.

Mastoid air cell system

This connects with the middle ear via the antrum. It provides a reservoir of air to balance vast changes in air pressure.

Eustachian tube

This tube provides a mechanism for the equalization of air pressure on either side of the TM (📖 see Fig. 6.1).

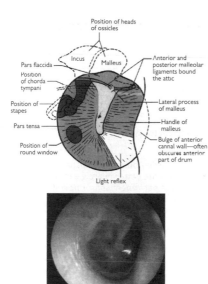

Fig. 6.1 Diagram of the tympanic membrane showing quadrants and what lies behind.

Congenital abnormalities of the middle ear

Congenital abnormalities of the middle ear are rare in isolation. Middle ear abnormalities are more common in association with microtia.

However, abnormalities of the ossicular chain can occur in isolation.

Signs and symptoms

- Conductive hearing loss never more than 60dB
- Normal tympanogram (or type A)

Management

- Diagnosis is usually carried out by a tympanotomy.
- If the abnormality is in the better hearing ear, use a hearing aid. Surgery carries a higher risk of permanent sensorineural loss.
- If the abnormality is in the worse hearing ear then consider a tympanotomy after a trial of a hearing aid.

Acute otitis media (📖 see Fig. 6.2)

This is a very common condition. Almost everyone will suffer with acute otitis media during their lifetime. Signs and symptoms may include a preceding URTI, severe and progressive otalgia, or a discharge—this is usually associated with a resolution of the otalgia.

A diagnosis is made by taking a history, examining the tympanic membrane, and taking the patient's temperature.

Treatment for acute otitis media is controversial. Systematic review suggests treatment with analgesia only. However, these reviews may have included a high proportion of viral ear infections where antibiotics would not be expected to be useful.

Management
- Give analgesia in all cases.
- Give oral antibiotics for one week such as co-amoxiclav PO.
- Warn the patient that the discharge may continue for 1 week.
- When the infection has resolved always check that the tympanic membrane has returned to normal.

Recurrent infections of the middle ear

These must be differentiated from one persisting infection. Treat any acute infections actively as above. If the patient has more than five infections in 6 months, then consider alternative treatment such as grommet insertion or a prolonged course of antibiotics.

Treatment
- **Medical**—consider prophylaxis with trimethoprim (TMP)/ sulfamethoxazole (SMX) syrup—2mg/kg TMP and 10mg/kg SMX as a single nightly dose PO for 3 months.
- **Surgical**—if there is an effusion or glue ear has been present for longer than 3 months consider grommet insertion ± adenoidectomy.
- **All treatment needs monitoring**—use an infection diary to record episodes of infection pre- and post-treatment.

Caution

Acute otitis media is often misdiagnosed. Children with nocturnal earache often have glue ear/Eustachian tube dysfunction. The tympanic membrane may be red or infected but there is no discharge and the pain resolves very quickly upon waking.

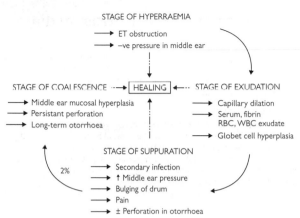

Fig. 6.2 Acute otitis media stages.

Complications of acute otitis media

Chronic infection

An infection may persist and become chronic. This may be due to resistant bacteria. Use a broad-spectrum antibiotic such as ciprofloxacin.

Consider myringotomy for the relief of symptoms or to obtain microbiological information.

Facial nerve palsy

10% of people have a dehiscent facial nerve—when the bony covering is absent over the nerve. This may result in a facial nerve irritation and palsy secondary to the middle ear inflammation.

The patient must be admitted to hospital and given IV antibiotics, e.g. cefuroxime. Also consider steroid therapy, prednisolone 1 mg/kg per day, if there is total facial paralysis, to be continued for 1 week.

Consider myringotomy and grommet insertion if the condition fails to resolve in 24h.

Acute mastoiditis

This is an infection of the mastoid air cells which will lead to a severe earache with tenderness, swelling, and redness behind the pinna. The pinna may also be pushed forwards, making it look more prominent.

Chronic perforation of the tympanic membrane

Repeated infections which perforate the tympanic membrane can lead to chronic perforation. The ear discharge may then present without pain.

Sensorineural hearing loss (SNHL)

Rarely, toxins can spread to the inner ear to produce a sensorineural hearing loss.

Vertigo

Infection near the lateral semicircular canal can produce a para-labyrinthitis. This can cause a spectrum of vestibular disturbance, ranging from mild unsteadiness to disabling vertigo.

Glue ear/otitis media with effusion

Glue ear is caused by a combination of exposure to infection and a non-functioning Eustachian tube. Almost 8 out of 10 children will have glue ear at some time during childhood. The incidence of glue ear decreases with age as the immune system develops and the Eustachian tube function improves.

The signs and symptoms of glue ear can include: decreased hearing, recurrent ear infections, poor speech development, failing performance at school, and, sometimes, antisocial behaviour.

Risk factors
- Smoking parents
- Bottle feeding
- Day-care nursery
- Cleft palate
- Atopy

Investigations
- Full history and examination (including the palate)
- Age appropriate audiometry and tympanometry

Management
This depends on a balance of:
- **Social factors**—more urgent action is needed if the family is unlikely to re-attend for further appointments
- **Hearing disability**—how the child is coping with their hearing problem socially and at school is more important than the actual level of hearing loss
- **Appearance of tympanic membranes**—if there is gross retraction, intervention may be needed to avoid retraction pocket formation

Treatment
There are three options:
- **Watchful waiting**—this should apply to all patients for 3 months as glue ear will resolve in 50% of cases
- **Hearing aid**—there is a window of opportunity at 4–8 years of age. It is non-invasive, but may lead to teasing at school
- **Insertion of grommets**—short general anaesthetic ± adenoidectomy

Chronic suppurative otitis media without cholesteatoma

This common condition is associated with Eustachian tube dysfunction with or without an infection in the mastoid.

As with other ear diseases, its prevalence continues despite antibiotics.

The signs and symptoms of chronic suppurative otitis media may include persistent recurrent otorrhoea, perforation in the tympanic membrane (usually central), and no cholesteatoma present.

Risk factors
- Smoking patient
- Smoking parents
- Acute otitis media
- Decreased immunity

Investigations
- Full history and ENT examination
- Microscopy of the eardrum with aural toilet
- Swab for microbiology

Management
- Give appropriate topical and systemic antibiotics based on the swab result. The condition may settle with antibiotics and water precautions.
- Perform regular cleaning of the ear using microsuction—aural toilet
- Persistent infections may need surgery.
- Myringoplasty (□ see p. 104).
- Cortical mastoidectomy (□ see p. 104).

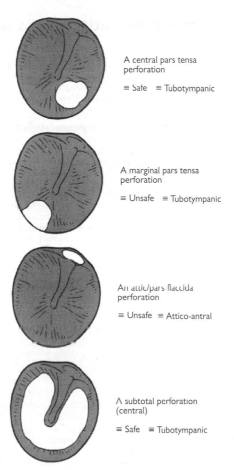

A central pars tensa
perforation

≡ Safe   ≡ Tubotympanic

A marginal pars tensa
perforation

≡ Unsafe   ≡ Tubotympanic

An attic/pars flaccida
perforation

≡ Unsafe   ≡ Attico-antral

A subtotal perforation
(central)

≡ Safe   ≡ Tubotympanic

Fig. 6.3 Diagram showing sites of perforations.

Chronic suppurative otitis media with cholesteatoma

This is often divided into congenital and acquired forms of the condition:
- Congenital cholesteatoma results from an abnormal focus of squamous epithelium in the middle ear space, i.e. a dermoid.
- Acquired cholesteatoma most often results from chronic Eustachian tube dysfunction.

It was hoped that the incidence of this condition would have changed with the advent of antibiotics. Unfortunately, the disease continues and can present at any age. Signs and symptoms may include recurrent otitis media with a mucopurulent discharge, hearing loss, facial nerve palsy, and vertigo.

Development of a cholesteatoma

Prolonged low middle ear pressure allows for the development of a pars flaccida retraction pocket. As this enlarges its neck becomes small compared to the sac itself. Initially, squamous epithelium migrates out of the sac with ease, but as it enlarges the squamous epithelium builds up and can no longer escape. If infection supervenes on the impacted squamous epithelium/keratin, then lytic enzymes are released causing destruction of local structures.

Management

- Aural toilet
- Microscopy and suction clearance
- Topical antibiotic/steroid (e.g. Sofradex®) drops for 10 days
- Review under the microscope after 1 month
- Audiometry
- CT scan of the temporal bone to look for pneumatization of mastoid or erosion of scutum (outer attic wall).

Management

This depends on the age and fitness of the patient, which ear is affected, the patient's wishes, and their ability to tolerate ear toilet.
- **Prophylaxis**—this is a controversial treatment where early retraction pockets are treated by inserting a grommet to reverse the development of a cholesteatoma.
- **Early retraction pocket**—attempting to clean the pocket and remove keratin. GA may be required. Maintenance of a cleaned pocket can be undertaken by an aural care specialist nurse.
- **Established non-cleaning pocket**—where the worst hearing ear is affected, surgery will usually be required to reduce the risk of intracerebral complications (⊞ see 'Surgery for CSOM', p. 104).

Follow-up

These patients are at risk of recurrence and therefore they need careful follow-up.

Complications of CSOM

These are related to local and distant effects of cholesteatoma (📖 see Fig. 6.4).

Local effects

- **Conductive hearing loss**—as the retracted attic segment of the eardrum lies against the long process of the incus, it interferes with its already tenuous blood supply. The incus initially thins then loses its attachment to the stapes. The cholesteatoma can bridge this gap and temporarily improve the conductive loss.
- **Sensorineural hearing loss**—the toxic effect of the local infection can cause a sensorineural hearing loss.
- **Vertigo**—may be due either to a para-labyrinthitis causing an irritative vestibulopathy, or it may be the result of erosion into the lateral semicircular canal—causing a fistula.
- **Facial nerve dysfunction**—if a dehiscence exists, infection can produce a direct irritation of the nerve. The cholesteatoma may also directly erode the bony covering of the facial nerve.
- **Mastoiditis**—a chronic infection may lead to mastoiditis.

Distant effects

- **Meningitis**—the roof of the middle ear is also the floor of the middle cranial fossa. A thin plate of bone separates the middle ear from the meninges in this area. This can be eroded by an extensive cholesteatoma, with a spread of infection to the meninges.
- **Cerebral abscess**—spread of infection can lead to abscess formation which can progress to the temporal lobe.
- **Lateral sinus thrombosis**—the lateral sinus is one of the relations of the mastoid air cell system. Infection can spread to the lateral sinus, causing local thrombosis. This in turn can lead to hydrocephalus.
- **Bezold's abscess**—infection from the mastoid spreads through the mastoid tip and travels under the sternomastoid, it then points in the neck anterior to the muscle.
- **Citelli's abscess**—infection spreads medially from the mastoid tip to collect in the digastric fossa.

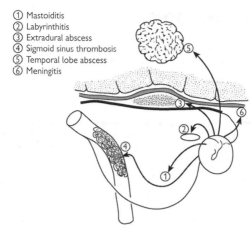

1. Mastoiditis
2. Labyrinthitis
3. Extradural abscess
4. Sigmoid sinus thrombosis
5. Temporal lobe abscess
6. Meningitis

Fig. 6.4 Routes of spread of infection from the middle ear.

Surgery for CSOM

In the absence of cholesteatoma the surgical options are designed to repair the perforation of the tympanic membrane and remove the source of chronic infection, so making the ear safe. Repair of the tympanic membrane will make the ear waterproof and reduce any discharge.

Myringoplasty is the patching of the hole in the tympanic membrane using either temporalis fascia or tragal perichondrium. The graft is usually applied to the undersurface of the tympanic membrane under a general anaesthetic. Surface tension keeps it in place. The graft acts as a scaffold for the tympanic membrane to grow across. During the procedure the tympanic membrane is lifted up to facilitate access for graft placement and assessment of the middle ear and ossicular chain. The procedure has an 85–90% success rate. Revision surgery carries an equally high success rate. Persistent failures are likely to be due to poor Eustachian tube function.

Cortical mastoidectomy is occasionally performed in conjunction with myringoplasty. The mastoid cavity is entered via a postauricular incision and the air cells drilled away to form a continuous cavity which joins the middle ear space at the mastoid antrum. The rationale for this approach is to remove any pockets of diseased mastoid mucosa or sepsis which can perpetuate the discharging ear.

In the presence of cholesteatoma different surgical criteria apply:
• Make the ear safe
• Make the ear clean and dry
• Restore hearing function

The ear is deemed unsafe until the full extent of the cholesteatomatous disease is known. Even CT can be misleading when it comes to evaluating the extent of the disease. Side effects from the spread of infection can be serious, e.g. meningitis, cerebral abscess (□ see 'Complications of CSOM, p. 102). The whole cholesteatoma should be removed. Any surgery performed must try and preserve as much of a normal ear structure as possible and should facilitate the natural self-cleaning mechanism of the external ear.

The function of the ear can be addressed by restoring the integrity of the tympanic membrane and ensuring that the ossicular chain is intact and functioning.

Surgical clearance of the disease should not be compromised by attempts at hearing preservation.

Atticotomy here the cholesteatoma just occupies the attic region of the middle ear space. Removal of the cholesteatoma can be accomplished by saucerizing the superior margin of the tympanic bony annulus and grafting the TM defect.

Atticoantrostomy involves more extensive removal, including the opening of the mastoid antrum.

Modified radical mastoidectomy cholesteatoma is usually extensive and travels back into the mastoid. The cholesteatoma is removed and followed back into the mastoid air cell system. The mastoid system is then joined to the EAC by drilling away the posterior bony canal wall of the EAC. This creates a common cavity of EAC and mastoid. The cavity is lined with temporalis fascia which will mucosalize with time. The ear is made safe as any recurrences can be seen using a microscope. Disease will travel outward along the path of least resistance rather than eroding through bone to the cranial cavity. The cavity usually does not stay clean on its own. Annual suction clearance is usually required. Larger cavities have more problems.

Combined approach tympanoplasty (CAT) is an alternative approach for the larger cholesteatoma. The cholesteatoma is removed by surgery via the EAC and via a mastoid approach. The posterior EAC wall is kept intact to minimize the need for lifelong cavity cleaning and to improve the auditory characteristics of the ear, which are believed to be better with an intact EAC. The drawback is the need for re-operation in approximately a year to check for any recurrent disease.

Ossiculoplasty is the reconstruction of the ossicular chain, using incus, cartilage, or prostheses. In general, the more of the normal ossicular chain that is present the easier it is to achieve a good hearing result. Presence of a normal stapes superstructure and short malleus to stapes head distance are thought to be good prognostic factors. Overall, hearing results show that 50% improve audiologically.

Otosclerosis

Here new bone is formed around the stapes footplate, which leads to its fixation and consequent conductive hearing loss. This condition is believed to start at a single focus in the lateral wall of the middle ear space near the oval window and stapes footplate. It manifests as slowly progressive hearing loss, usually beginning in the patient's twenties. There is usually a family history of the condition. The patient may have difficulty hearing when chewing and may have problems with quiet conversations. Some 69–80% of patients have tinnitus. Dizziness is rarely caused by this condition. Accelerated progression is often seen during pregnancy.

In its early stages the lesion is 'spongiotic'. Later, this spongiosis becomes sclerosis, or a combination of these two abnormal bone types. Later still, osteocytes at the edge of the lesion extend into the bone, surrounding the central vascular spaces. Stapes fixation occurs when the annular ligament or stapes footplate becomes involved. Spread to the cochlea produces high-tone sensorineural hearing loss.

Incidence
- The female to male ratio is 2:1.
- 6.4% of temporal bones have evidence of otosclerosis.
- 0.3% of the population have a clinical manifestation of the disease.
- The condition is bilateral in 70% of patients.
- 50% of patients with otosclerosis have a family history.

Investigations
- Check for a normal mobile intact tympanic membrane.
- Look for 'Schwartzes sign'—flamingo pink blush of the TM seen at otoscopy anterior to the position of the oval window. Believed to be due to increased vascular supply to the otospongiotic focus.
- Perform pure tone audiometry. This shows conductive hearing loss (CHL) often with the typical Carhart's notch (Fig. 6.5).
- Check for absent stapedial reflex.
- Consider a CT scan—this may help to exclude other bony abnormalities of the middle ear causing ossicular fixation.

Differential diagnosis
Paget's disease—this is the only other bony lesion which involves the middle ear. Here there is increased alkaline phosphatase and a mixed hearing loss.

Osteogenesis imperfecta—(also known as Van der Hoeve syndrome) leads to mixed hearing loss with blue sclera. There is frequently a history of multiple bony fractures.

Treatment
The options are:
- No treatment
- Hearing aid
- Surgery—stapedectomy after a 3-month trial of a hearing aid

Patient selection for surgery

Because one of the complications of stapedectomy is complete SNHL careful patient selection is vital.

- Surgery is usually only performed on the worse hearing ear.
- Sensorineural hearing loss in the contralateral ear is a contraindication.
- If there is tympanic membrane perforation, this will necessitate a myringoplasty first.
- Active infection must be controlled prior to surgery to prevent any potential infection of the prosthesis or, worse still, spread of infection to the inner ear.

Cochlear otosclerosis

This is due to the spread of the otosclerotic process to the basal turn of the cochlea. Treatment with sodium fluoride helps to reduce the abnormal bone metabolism and so stabilizes hearing loss.

Monitor with serial pure tone audiograms.

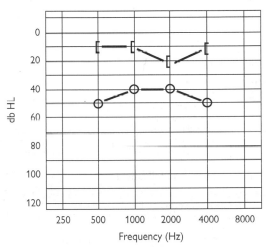

Fig. 6.5 Pure tone audiometry showing conductive hearing loss typical Cahart's notch.

Trauma and neoplasia

Acoustic trauma

Loud noise can produce direct traumatic effects on the middle ear.
(📖 see 'Noise-induced hearing loss', p. 118).

Head injury

Direct blows to the head can produce:
- A temporal bone fracture
- A haemotympanum—blood in the middle ear
- Ossicular chain disruption
- Rarely, cochlear concussion can produce an SNHL

Management

Patients with severe trauma may present late to ENT, as they usually
have more pressing management priorities. Treat the patient's head injury
and check for a cervical spine injury. Perform otoscopy and look for CSF
otorrhoea. Check the facial nerve function.

Hearing assessment

- A tuning fork test will distinguish CHL from SNHL.
- Pure tone audiogram will confirm the tuning fork findings and will
  quantify any hearing defect.

Treatment

- **SNHL**—consider steroids: prednisolone 1mg/kg OD for one week if
  no contraindications. Follow with serial audiograms.
- **CHL**—no immediate treatment. Review in OPD in 6 weeks. The
  haemotympanum will have resolved. Re-test the patient's hearing. If
  CHL persists check the tympanogram to ensure that there is no glue
  ear and consider tympanotomy with ossicular reconstruction.

Pens, cotton buds, and lollysticks

If these objects are inserted into the EAC, they rarely reach the
eardrum. They usually impact on the skin of the EAC and tear it,
causing bleeding. Careful examination with the otoscope can usually
identify this problem.

Traumatic perforations of the TM usually heal spontaneously. Treat
haemotympanum and possible ossicular dislocation as above.

Neoplasia

Benign and malignant tumours involving the middle ear space can occur,
but these are very rare.

The inner ear

Structure and function of the inner ear

The inner ear can be divided into two parts—the cochlea and the vestibular system (Fig. 7.1).

The cochlea

This is the organ of sound transduction. The cochlea is a coiled helix, and is encased in hard bone of the petrous temporal bone.

The specialized structure of the cochlea turns sound waves into electrochemical signals which pass to the brain.

The cochlea has a tonotopic representation—this means that different areas are frequency-specific. High frequencies are dealt with at the start or at the base of the cochlea. Low tones are dealt with at the cochlear apex. (□ See Fig. 7.2 for a cross-section of the cochlea.)

The neurological pathway to the auditory cortex is best remembered by using the E COLI mnemonic:

E Eighth nerve
C Cochlear nucleus
O Superior olive
L Lateral lemniscus
I Inferior colliculus

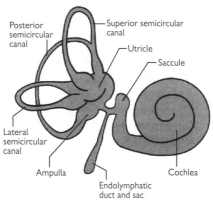

Fig. 7.1 Diagram of the inner ear.

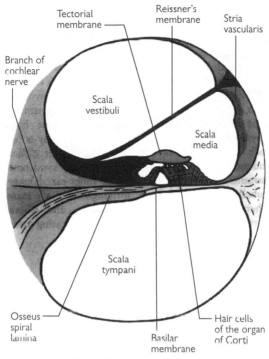

Fig. 7.2 Cross-section of the cochlea.

Vestibular system

The vestibular system functions to provide information to the brain about angular and linear acceleration of the head. It is also encased in the petrous temporal bone.

Five separate neuroepithelial elements work in combination to provide this information: 3 semicircular canals, the utricle, and the saccule.

The semicircular canals are paired to provide complimentary information about the direction of travel.

The inferior and superior vestibular nerves pass the information to the brain.

The ultrastructure of these neuroepithelial elements is shown in Figs 7.3 and 7.4.

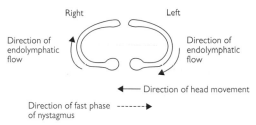

Fig. 7.3 Paired motion of the semicircular canals.

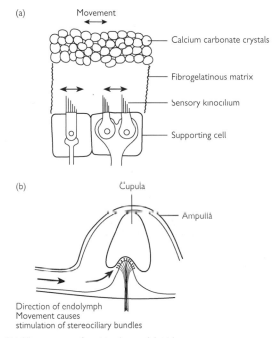

Fig. 7.4 Ultrastructure of semicircular canals/utricle.

Hearing loss

The aetiology of hearing loss can be determined by careful consideration of the patient's history, a clinical examination, and the findings of special investigations.

The age of onset of the patient's hearing loss is important, as is any family history of hearing loss. Careful consideration of a patient's pregnancy and perinatal history are also important.

Examination

This will aim to discover any congenital abnormality or inherited syndrome in which hearing loss may play a part (Table 7.1).

Ears	Preauricular pits present?
	Shape and location of the pinnae
	Size of the EAC
	Appearance of the TM
Eyes	Eyebrows
	Interpupillary distance
	Colour of the iris
	External ocular movements
	Appearance of the fundus
	Retinal pigment
Face	Shape
	Symmetry
Skin	Texture
	Pigmentation
Extremities	Shape of the fingers and toes
	Carrying angle

Investigations

These should aim to confirm and assess the extent of the patient's hearing loss and to look for any evidence of an inherited condition:
- Audiogram
- Radiology
- Blood tests:
- U+Es
  - glucose
  - TFTs
  - ECG
  - cytogenetics

Specialist opinions

You may need to consult an ophthalmologist and/or a clinical geneticist.

Table 7.1 Classification of patients presenting with hearing loss

Non-hereditary	Hereditary
Presbyacusis	Syndromic
Noise-induced hearing loss	Non-syndromic
Idiopathic sudden hearing loss	
Autoimmune hearing loss	
Vascular causes	
Ototoxicity	
Non-organic hearing loss	

Presbyacusis

This term describes a decreased peripheral auditory sensitivity. It is usually age-related, and affects men more than women.

Signs and symptoms

This condition shows itself as bilateral, progressive, symmetrical sensorineural hearing loss, with no history of noise exposure. The patient may have poor speech discrimination compared with the audiogram. Decreasing central auditory discrimination leads to phonemic regression.

Investigations

- Otoscopy
- Pure tone audiogram (Fig. 7.5)

Types of presbyacusis

Based on the shape of the audiogram and the histological site of loss, presbyacusis can be subdivided into the following subtypes:

- **Sensory presbyacusis**—steep-sloping audiogram above speech frequency. It starts in mid-life so speech discrimination is preserved. Degeneration in the Organ of Corti.
- **Neural presbyacusis**—down-sloping, high-frequency loss. Flatter than sensory presbyacusis. Thought to be 1st order neuron loss. Disproportionate discrimination score.
- **Strial presbyacusis**—flat audiogram. Good discrimination.
- **Cochlear conductive/indeterminate presbyacusis**—down-sloping audiogram. Increasing stiffness of the basilar membrane.
- **Central presbyacusis**—loss of GABA in the inferior colliculus.
- **Middle ear ageing**—loosening of ligaments or ossicular articulation problem.

Management

The patient may be given counselling and advice about hearing loss, and given a hearing aid where the symptoms are troublesome.

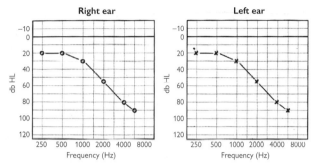

Fig. 7.5 Investigation of presbyacusis: pure tone audiogram for (a) right ear; (b) left ear.

Noise-induced hearing loss

This is defined as damage to the inner ear caused by exposure to loud noise. There is a relationship between the volume of sound and its duration which causes damage. Eight hours of exposure to a sound level of 85dB usually causes damage. Louder sounds will cause damage at shorter exposure times.

Acoustic trauma is caused by sounds greater than 180dB. Rupture of the tympanic membrane and ossicular fracture may occur.

Signs and symptoms

The patient will usually present with bilateral and symmetrical hearing loss. There may be a noise-induced temporary threshold shift (TTS)—for example, hearing may improve over the weekend if the problem is noise at work. The patient may have difficulty hearing in background noise or they may have tinnitus.

Investigations

Use audiometry. For a typical pattern 📖 see Fig. 7.6.

Pathology

Hearing loss is greatest in the 3–6kHz region of the cochlea. Below 2kHz the acoustic reflex is protective. Since EAC resonant frequency is 1–4kHz, energy delivered at these frequencies is greater. The actual loss of cochlear cells occurs where noise damage is greatest. Outer hair cells lose rigidity and the stereocilia fuse.

Management

Consider the following to prevent further noise damage:
- Health and safety at work
- Provision of ear defenders
- Routine hearing screening for occupations at risk

For established damage consider:
- Hearing aids
- Counselling for tinnitus

Rifle shooting

This will sometimes result in an asymmetrical SNHL with the noise-damaged pattern. When firing a rifle, one ear is nearer to the gun barrel. If the patient is right handed, their left ear is most affected as it is nearer to the barrel of the gun.

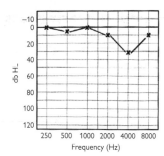

Fig. 7.6 Audiogram of noise damage.

Idiopathic sudden hearing loss

(📖 See 'Sudden-onset hearing loss', p. 376.)

Usually defined as the loss of 30dB or more over three contiguous frequencies on an audiogram. Sudden loss can be immediate, waking up with a loss, or having a progressive loss over several days.

Annual incidence is 5 per 100 000 of the population, but this is only an estimate.

- Unilateral loss common
- Bilateral sudden loss 1%
- Male and female of equal occurrence
- Median age 40 years

Aetiology

- Vascular disease
- Viral infection
- Autoimmune hearing loss
- Endolymphatic hydrops
- Neurological conditions, e.g. multiple sclerosis

Investigations

- Full blood count (FBC)
- Erythrocyte sedimentation rate (ESR) and C-reactive protein (CRP)
- Urea and electrolytes (U+Es)
- Fasting glucose
- Thyroid function tests (TFTs)
- Lipid profile
- Clotting studies
- Autoimmune profile
- MRI scan to exclude acoustic neuroma (3% of acoustic neuromas present with sudden hearing loss)

Audiological investigations

- PTA
- Tympanometry
- ABR or OAEs if non-organic loss suspected

Treatment

(📖 see 'Sudden-onset hearing loss', p. 376)

Prognosis

60% show at least some sign of recovery.

Autoimmune ear disease

Autoimmune ear disease is classified as either organ-specific, or as a systemic disease.

Organ-specific

Vestibuloauditory autoimmunity or evidence of cell-mediated immunity against inner ear antigens.

Systemic disease

Hearing loss may occur as part of a recognized systemic autoimmune disease. Common diseases which have auditory vestibular involvement are shown opposite.

Patients with autoimmune ear disease are usually middle-aged and are more likely to be male than female.

Signs and symptoms

- Bilateral unexplained SNHL
- May complain of fluctuant dizziness or Ménière-like syndrome with aural fullness
- Rapidly progressive hearing loss over days or weeks
- Associated VIIth nerve palsy
- Normal otoscopic examination
- Coexistent systemic immune disease

Investigations

Take a full history and give a full otoneurological examination, including a pure tone audiogram. Perform an MRI scan to exclude acoustic neuroma with unilateral presentation.

Carry out the following blood tests:
- Antigen-specific antibodies
- Antigen non-specific antibodies
- Acute-phase reactants
- Lyme titres

Treatment

Treatment should be given under the guidance of neurotolgist and/or a rheumatologist.

Give steroids such as prednisolone 1mg/kg per day PO, **or** consider steroid-sparing alternatives:
- Cyclophosphamide
- Methotrexate
- Plasmapheresis

The following conditions are thought to have an autoimmune basis and can cause hearing loss:

Polyarteritis nodosa

This condition affects the small and medium arteries. There is a rare association with an inner ear hearing loss.

Cogan's syndrome

This is a non-syphilitic interstitial keratitis with vestibuloauditory dysfunction. It presents with photophobia and lacrimation 1–6 months before vestibuloauditory symptoms develop.

Atypical Cogan's

This interstitial keratitis develops 1–2 years before auditory vestibular problems.

Wegener's granulomatosis

This is a necrotizing granulomatous vasculitis of the lower and upper respiratory tract which also affects the kidneys causing focal necrotizing glomerulonephritis. Some 90% of patients have a sensorineural hearing loss, and 20% have a conductive hearing loss with effusion.
cANCA-positive 90%.

Relapsing polychondritis

In this condition, a giant cell arteritis and systemic vasculitis cause recurrent episodes of inflammatory necrosis. There is a raised ESR and a false-positive syphillis serology (VDRL).

Rheumatoid arthritis

RA is a very common disease with characteristic arthropathy.

Ototoxicity

Drugs can damage the cochlea and vestibular system. It is worth taking a careful drug history, as a wide range of drugs can cause symptoms. Cross-check with the *BNF* for side-effects.

Aminoglycoside antibiotics

These antibiotics have a narrow therapeutic index and can cause damage to the inner ear. Common side effects are drug-induced vestibular symptoms and hearing loss.

Patients requiring parenteral aminoglycoside antibiotics should have the plasma levels of the drug monitored during therapy. Local policy varies; often trough levels of antibiotic are used to determine future dose levels.

Topical antibiotics

Most topical antibiotics available contain an aminoglycoside antibiotic. These drugs are experimentally ototoxic in guinea pigs and other animals. They are believed to enter the inner ear through the round window membrane causing direct ototoxic effects. Drug data sheets also warn of the risks of using these preparations when there are grommets *in situ* or where there is a perforation of the TM.

Short courses of these antibiotics—less than 10 days—are safe with perforations or grommets in the presence of infection. Oedema of the middle ear mucosa with a thickened round window membrane, limits the entry of antibiotic into the inner ear. *Untreated infection is a greater risk to hearing than the antibiotic.*

Therapeutic uses

Aminoglycosides can be used to treat patients with Ménière's disease by causing a vestibulopathy when instilled into the middle ear. Much higher doses are used compared with the standard drops.

Other drugs

Chemotherapy, especially cisplatin, induces SNHL.
Aspirin and erythromycin can cause a reversible SNHL. Patients present with tinnitus.

Hereditary hearing loss

Inherited hearing loss may be divided into syndromic and non-syndromic types. Non-syndromic hearing loss is most common, representing about two-thirds of cases.

As the loci of genes associated with hearing loss are identified, it becomes more obvious that the classifying of these conditions on syndromic basis may be misleading. Many patients with apparently non-syndromic heredi-tary hearing loss have the same gene alterations as their syndromic coun-terparts but are not phenotypically syndromic.

Other classifications of hereditary hearing loss are:

Genetics 📖 See Table 7.2

Age of onset Early (birth–age 2 years)

Known congenital
Suspected congenital

Delayed (3–20 years)
Adult (>21 years)

Hearing loss Sensorineural
Conductive
Mixed hearing loss

Laterality Unilateral/bilateral

Stability Stable
Fluctuating
Progressive

Frequencies Low (250–1kHz)
Medium (>1kHz–4kHz)
High (>4kHz)

Associations Radiological abnormalities
Vestibular dysfunction

Table 7.2 Genetic inheritance of hearing loss

Inheritance	Percentage	Condition
Autosomal recessive	60–70	Non-syndromic SNHL Pendred's Usher's Jervell–Lange-Nielsen
Autosomal dominant	20–25	Waardenburg's Branchio-oto-renal (BOR) syndrome Alport's
X-linked recessive	2–3	X-linked mixed hearing loss with stapes gusher
X-linked dominant	Uncertain	Alport's
Chromosomal	<1	
Mitochondrial	<1	
Multifactorial	Uncertain	

Syndromic hearing loss I

Goldenhar's syndrome (oculoauricularvertebral [OAV:] syndrome)

This is the most common syndrome, occurring in approximately 1 in 10 000 live births. It is sporadic, not caused by genetic inheritance.

Features of Goldenhar's syndrome (Fig. 7.7)

Face	25% marked asymmetry
	Maxilla and temporal bones reduced and flattened
	Hypoplasia/aplasia of mandible
Ear	Flattened helical rim
	Preauricular tags
	EAC atretic/small
Hearing loss	CHL
	SNHL 15%
Associations	Skeletal abnormalities c-spine/skull base
	Cleft lip/palate
	Velopharyngeal insufficiency
	Mental retardation 15%

Treacher Collins

Patients have a mandibulofacial dysostosis due to 1st/2nd branchial arch, groove, and pouch abnormalities. This is the commonest syndrome of hearing loss. 60% of cases are sporadic rather than genetic. This abnormality has been found to occur on gene 5q31–q34.

Features of Treacher Collins' syndrome (Fig. 7.8)

Face	Depressed cheeks
	Narrow midface
	Hypertelorism
Ear	Malformed cup-shaped pinnae
	Narrow EAC
	Malformed ossicles, cochlea, and labyrinth
Associations	Cleft palate
	Palatopharyngeal incompetence 30–40%
	Normal intelligence

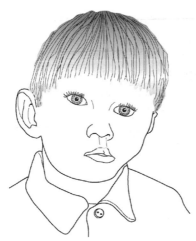

Fig. 7.7 Features of Goldenhar's syndrome.

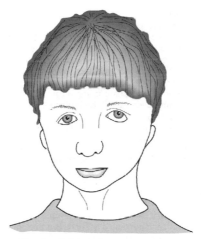

Fig. 7.8 Features of Treacher Collins syndrome.

Syndromic hearing loss II

Waardenburg's syndrome
2–5% of congenitally deaf children have Waardenburg's syndrome.

Features of Waardenburg's syndrome

Appearance	Dystopia canthorum in type 1
	Synophrys—confluent eyebrows 85% type 1
	Broad nasal root
	Heterochromia iridis (different colour irides)
	Sapphire eyes
	White forelock 30–40%
	Vitiligo
	Premature grey hair
Hearing loss	Congenital SNHL

20% of those with type 1 WS and 50% of those with type 2 have a hearing loss

50% of people with WS have normal hearing

Branchial–oto–renal syndrome (BOR)
In this rare condition there is an association of branchial fistulas/cysts with hearing problems and renal abnormalities.

Alport's syndrome
This is a rare hereditary progressive glomerulonephritis with SNHL. It presents as hearing loss and renal problems. There are six subtypes of Alport's syndrome classified by type of inheritance, age of onset of renal failure, presence of hearing loss, and ocular abnormalities.

The diagnosis of Alport's syndrome depends on three out of four of the following being found:
• Positive family history of haematuria and renal failure
• Electron microscopic evidence of glomerulonephritis on renal biopsy
• Characteristic ophthalmic signs
• Progressive high-frequency SNHL starting in childhood

Pendred's syndrome
This is a rare autosomal recessive condition where a non-toxic goitre is found in association with profound congenital SNHL.

It is associated with the Mondini deformity of the cochlea.

Jervell–Lange-Nielsen syndrome
In this condition SNHL is believed to be autosomal recessive. The abnormality is located on chromosome 11. There is a prolonged QT interval on ECG. Multiple syncopal episodes may occur from the age of 3–5 years onwards.

Usher's syndrome
This is an autosomal recessive condition consisting of retinitis pigmentosa and hearing impairment. There are three subtypes, with types I and II sufferers born deaf, and type III gradually becoming deaf.

Non-organic hearing loss (NOHL)

This describes a situation where a patient claims to have a hearing loss where none exists, or where a patient exaggerates a hearing loss which does exist.

A typical example may be a child who is having difficulties at school or at home, and who presents with a very poor hearing test result. Often the hearing loss documented on the audiogram will seem out of keeping with the child's participation in the consultation. Another example is a patient who is pursuing a claim for damages as a result of a hearing loss.

The clues to look for when diagnosing this condition are: concerns raised by the audiologist about inconsistent results, if there is litigation involved, or if the parent–child interaction is unusual.

Investigations

- Pure tone audiometry
- Tuning fork tests—Stenger test (📖 see 'Stenger test' below)
- Speech audiogram—more difficult to fabricate abnormal response
- Stapedial reflex testing
- Delayed speech feedback—the patient reads aloud and their speech is played into the affected ear. The playback is slightly delayed which will cause the patient to hesitate or stutter if they can hear
- Brainstem evoked auditory response—this is the 'gold standard' in litigation cases

Management

Careful handling of patients with non-organic hearing loss is required. It may be wise to suggest to affected children that you know their hearing is better, but don't be too confrontational. Bring them back for another audiogram and suggest that they try to be a little more accurate.

Litigation claims need more tact and multiple investigations before any confrontation.

Stenger test

Use two 512Hz tuning forks.

Step 1

The patient closes their eyes and the examiner stands behind.
The tuning fork is activated and placed at 5cm from each ear in turn.
The patient will hear the note in their good ear but deny hearing it in the non-hearing ear.

Step 2

- Both tuning forks are used without the patient realizing it.
- One is held 5cm from the ear with the alleged poor hearing. The other is held, at the same time, 15cm away from the good ear.
- The patient with NOHL will deny hearing any sound. The tuning fork held near the bad ear will mask the sound of the tuning fork near the good ear. However, the genuine patient will only hear the tuning fork near the good ear.

Labyrinthitis (vestibular neuronitis)

This presents as a sudden episode of vertigo in a previously well person. It is equally common in men and women, with the usual age of onset being 30–40 years. Attacks are usually single, but people may occasionally experience multiple attacks, and it can be recurrent. It normally lasts 1–2 days and improves over weeks. Vertigo is usually unilateral or, rarely, bilateral. Epidemics can occur in the spring or summer. There may be an associated URTI 2 weeks prior to the vertigo. It occasionally leaves a BPPV symptom complex.

Pathology
- Axonal loss—endoneurial fibrosis and atrophy of the nerve
- Suspected viral aetiology, e.g. rubeola, herpes simplex virus (HSV), reovirus, cytomegalovirus (CMV), influenza, and mumps

Signs and symptoms
- Nystagmus away from the affected side
- Quix test +ve (seated Romberg's test)

Investigations
- Pure tone audiograms
- ENG if there is clinical doubt about the diagnosis
- MRI if there is asymmetry or recurrent episodes

Treatment
- Vestibular suppressant for acute attack—prochlorperazine 5mg sub-buccal/12.5mg IM
- Steroids if SNHL—prednisolone 1mg/kg for 1 week
- Patients usually compensate well for this condition
- Vestibular rehabilitation—for patients who do not compensate
- Vestibular suppressants can delay recovery if abused

Decompensations

During recovery from labrynthitis (or other vertigo causes) patients may suffer shorter-lived episodes of vertigo which are less severe. These are thought to represent temporary failure of the brain to compensate. They usually diminish with time from the original sudden onset of vertigo.

Benign paroxysmal positional vertigo (BPPV)

This is the most common cause of peripheral vertigo. It usually starts around the age of 50 years. The patient experiences brief episodes of vertigo caused by changes in position. It is worse in the morning and the evening. This condition is believed to occur as a result of stimulation of the semicircular canals by otoliths which have become misplaced.

There are three typical patterns in benign paroxysmal positional vertigo:

- Acute form—resolves in 3 months
- Intermittent form—active and inactive periods over years
- Chronic form—has continuous symptoms over longer duration.

Investigations

- Full otoneurological examination
- Dix–Hallpike test (see below)
- Pure tone audiogram
- ENG—if there is diagnostic uncertainty
- MRI scan—if symptoms persistent for more than 3 months

Dix–Hallpike test

- Place the patient on the examining couch, positioned in such a way that when they lie back their head will be over the end of the bed.
- While the patient is sitting turn their head 30° towards the examiner. This leads to maximal stimulation of the posterior semicircular canal (PSCC) on lying down.
- Then ask the patient to lie down, looking at the examiner's nose. The examiner supports the head and allows the head to extend over the edge of the bed.
- A positive test results in rotatory nystagmus after a delay of 1–5s, which lasts for 10–30s. Reversal to the upright position changes the direction of the nystagmus.
- This process is fatiguable, and sensitivity of the test can be improved with Frenzel glasses which do not allow optic fixation.

Treatment

- **Fatiguing exercises**—if the patient has significant symptom-free episodes (🕮 see Fig. 7.9).
- **Epley manoeuvre**—can bring 90% relief if the patient has had symptoms for more than 3–4 weeks (🕮 see Fig. 7.10).
- **Surgery**—this is rare. A singular neurectomy may lead to SNHL in 10–20% of patients. A retrosigmoid vestibular nerve section carries a 1% mortality risk as the procedure involves craniotomy. A posterior canal occlusion via a mastoid operation will control the symptoms, but an SNHL may complicate 5% of cases.

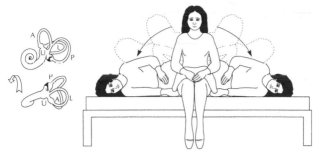

Fig. 7.9 Brandt–Daroff exercises.

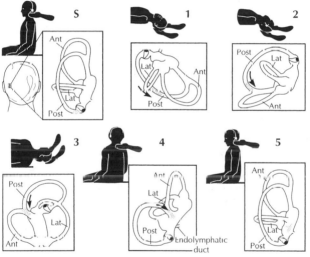

Fig. 7.10 Epley manoeuvre.

Ménière's disease/syndrome

Ménière's syndrome presents itself as increasing fullness in the ear and roaring tinnitus, giving a sensation of blocked hearing. An episode of vertigo may follow. Alternatively, there may be a sudden onset of vertigo with no warning (see Signs and symptoms below). Some 30–50% of people with Ménière's syndrome have bilateral symptoms within 3 years of presentation.

Presentation

Ménière's syndrome:
- Affects 50–150 people per 100 000 of the population
- Is more common in females than in males
- Usually occurs between the ages of 35 and 40 years

Causes

- Idiopathic—Ménière's disease
- Post-traumatic (head injury or ear surgery)
- Postinfectious delayed (e.g. mumps and measles)
- Late-stage syphilis
- Classical Cogan's
- Atypical Cogan's

Signs and symptoms

Of people with Ménière's disease:
- 42% have hearing loss alone
- 11% have vertigo alone
- 44% have vertigo and hearing loss
- 3% have tinnitus

Vertigo lasts more than 20 minutes and is associated with nausea, vomiting, and autonomic effects. Most episodes last 2–4 hours (although some last for more than 6 hours).

Horizontal or horizonto-rotatory nystagmus is always present.

The patient may experience disequilibrium after an attack of several days' duration.

A fluctuating SNHL is found in the early stages of the disease. Later, the hearing loss becomes permanent. The hearing may not change for some days after an attack.

Types of hearing loss

- Low-frequency SNHL
- Flat, moderately severe SNHL
- Bilateral SNHL with >25dB asymmetry

Poorly controlled patients have progressive hearing loss, stabilizing at 50–60dB.

Variant presentations of Ménière's disease
These include:
- Lermoyez variant—hearing improves with vertigo attacks
- Otolithic crisis of Tumarkin—patient has drop attacks with vertigo (decompression of saccule)
- Cochlear Ménière's—auditory symptoms only
- Vestibular Ménière's—vestibular symptoms only

Investigations
- Otoneurological examination
- Pure tone audiogram
- MRI scan if there is asymmetry
- Autoantibodies—ESR, antinuclear antibody (ANA), RhF, IgGs
- Echocochleography (ECoG)—this test involves placing a recording electrode either in the EAC or through the tympanic membrane to rest against the promontory of the cochlea. Sound is then applied to the test ear and the electrical activity in the ear is documented. Several components can be identified and measured. An increased ratio of the summating potential compared to the action potential (>0.4) suggests hydrops (Fig. 7.11).

Pathology
On sectioning the inner ear in affected patients, the scala media is found to be expanded, as if there has been too much pressure in the endolymph. This is known as 'endolymphatic hydrops'.

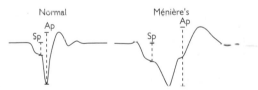

Fig. 7.11 Diagram of ECoG waveform.

Treatment of Ménière's disease

Medical management
- Prophylaxis
  - no added salt in diet
  - caffeine avoidance
  - betahistine 16mg tds PO
  - bendroflumethiazide 2.5 mg od
- For acute attacks of vertigo—prochlorperazine 5 mg sublingual or buccal
- Six-monthly review with symptom diary recording vertigo 'spinning' episodes and the length of each episode.

Surgical intervention
Patients whose symptoms are not improved by maximum medical therapy will require active intervention. 📖 See Table 7.3.

> ### Principles of intervention
>
> All treatments balance the control of vertiginous episodes with the risk of hearing loss and the associated morbidity of the procedure. Treatment should not be undertaken for non-vertiginous symptoms. Care should be undertaken when dealing with the better hearing ear.

Factors affecting the choice of intervention
- Patient choice
- Surgeon's preference
- Cost of treatment
- Hearing level in affected ear
- Patient fitness

Measuring success
Guidelines from the American Academy of Otorhinolaryngologists and Head and Neck Surgeons (AOHNS) measure success by comparing number of vertiginous episodes in the 6 months prior to treatment with the number of episodes 6 months after treatment and following up for 2 years.

Table 7.3 Comparison of treatments for Ménière's disease

Procedure	Indications	Control of vertigo (%)	Risk of hearing loss	Cost	Risk
Transtympanic gentamicin injection	Hearing loss <50dB	85	5%	Low	Low
Endolymphatic sac decompression	Fluctuating SNHL	65	<5%	Medium	Low
Total labyrinthectomy	Hearing loss >60dB	95	Total loss	Medium	Low–medium
Vestibular nerve section	Long-standing disease. Hearing loss <50dB	90	<5%	High	Medium

Vascular causes of inner ear dysfunction

Vascular occlusion of the labyrinthine artery can cause the sudden onset of vertigo and hearing loss. This occlusion leads to widespread necrosis of membranous structures and labyrinthitis ossificans. The patient may have a prior history of transient ischaemic attacks (TIAs)—62% of TIA patients have episodic vertigo. Compensation usually occurs in 4–6 months.

Occlusion of anterior vestibular artery
- Produces hearing loss and vertigo.
- As the posterior circulation remains intact, the patient may simply present with a BPPV-like symptom complex.

Recurrent vestibulopathy/vascular loop syndrome
- Some 7% of vertigo patients experience this syndrome. It is believed to occur as a result of an abnormally placed blood vessel impacting upon the vestibular nerve in the internal auditory meatus.
- Females with this syndrome outnumber males by a 2:1 ratio. The optimum age is 35–55 years old.
- The patient has usually had symptoms of episodic vertigo for 3 years at presentation; 80% have had episodic vertigo within the previous year; and 10% have BPPV.
- PTA shows a high-frequency loss in 50% of patients and a middle frequency loss in 20%.
- The resulting histological abnormality is axonal loss and endoneurial fibrosis.

Features
- Look for spontaneous nystagmus
- Non-classical Dix–Hallpike test— no fatigue

Investigations
- Pure tone audiograms
- MRI/MRA

Treatment
- Vestibular suppressants—prochlorperazine 5mg sublingual/buccal tds for vertigo.
- Consider microvascular nerve decompression.

Temporal bone fractures

These require significant force and therefore result from a serious head injury. Patients with this injury often present late to the ENT surgeon. Other injuries usually take precedence.

Types of fracture

These fractures are described according to their orientation to the axis of the temporal bone. Most fractures are complex and do not fit with the standard patterns:

- 80% are longitudinal(fracture line lateral to medial)
- 20% are transverse (fracture line anterior to posterior)

Management

Treat head injury and other trauma according to the Advanced Trauma Life Support (ATLS) protocol.

As part of a secondary survey:

- Examine behind ears for bruises (Battle's sign)
- Look for periorbital bruising (raccoon sign)
- Examine for nystagmus and record degree. (See opposite for classification of nystagmus.)
- Examine EAC for blood/CSF
- Examine TM for disruption of annulus
- Perform tuning fork tests (Weber and Rinne)
- Test facial nerve function

Investigations

- Audiometry
- CT scan—often a head injury scan will not show a fracture.
- CT scan of the temporal bone with fine-cut bony windows gives the best diagnostic information and prognosis for hearing loss.

Classical pattern of temporal bone fractures

Longitudinal fracture—often caused by lateral blow to head

- Blood in EAC
- Haemotympanum
- Disruption of annulus
- SNHL only temporary
- Facial nerve injury uncommon (20%)—it can occur if not exactly longitudinal. Statistically this type of fracture causes more facial nerve palsies. Usually damaged in horizontal part of the nerve
- CSF otorrhoea temporary phenomenon.

Transverse fracture—often caused by parietal or occipital blow

- EAC normal
- Haemotympanum can occur but not common
- SNHL permanent
- Facial nerve injury in 50%
- Vertigo and nystagmus IIIrd degree

Priorities in management

- **Manage facial nerve injury**—📖 see 'Facial palsy or VIIth nerve palsy', p. 378.
- **Managing CHL**—haemotympanum will resolve in 4 weeks.
  Persistent problems afterwards may be due to ossicular discontinuity.
  Tympanotomy and exploration of middle ear may be required.
- **Managing vertigo**—vestibular rehabilitation under guidance of physiotherapist.
- **Managing BPPV**—📖 see 'Benign paroxysmal positional vertigo', p. 136.
- **Managing SNHL**—rehabilitation with appropriate hearing aids.

Classification of nystagmus

Nystagmus is an irregular movement of the eyes characterized by a slow tracking phase followed by a fast corrective phase in the opposite direction. It is described in terms of its fast-phase movement. The direction of movement can be classified into horizontal (often peripheral vestibular system), vertical (usually CNS disease), and rotatory (BPPV). It is further classified into degrees by the direction of eye movement which causes the nystagmus to be evident:

- Ist degree—only when looking in direction of fast beat phase of nystagmus
- IInd degree—looking in direction of fast beat and straight ahead
- IIIrd degree—looking in all directions

Hearing rehabilitation

Rehabilitation of hearing is important to restore both social and psychological health.

Controversy exists especially in parts of the deaf community about the most appropriate forms of rehabilitation. Children who are born profoundly deaf are often encouraged to communicate using sign language rather than consider options such as cochlear implantation. Ultimately personal choice plays a role in selecting these options.

Forms of rehabilitation
- Sign language
- Lip reading
- Conventional hearing aids
- Bone-anchored hearing aids
- Cochlear implantation
- Brainstem auditory implants

Conventional hearing aids

The essential components of a hearing aid are a microphone to capture sound, a signal processor/amplifier which can be programmed to amplify sounds to fit the hearing loss profile of the patient, and a speaker system. Aids can be classified into their appearance and where they are to be located:
- **Body worn**—easy to use for elderly patients with limited dexterity, but they are obvious.
- **BTE or behind-the-ear aids**—the commonest type of aid and a good balance between practicality and appearance.
- **ITE or in-the-ear aids**—this aid sits in the conchal bowl and offers superior cosmesis over the preceding aids. May have limited power for severe loss.
- **CIC or completely-in-the-canal aids**—cosmetically the best, but can be limited on power.

BAHA or bone-anchored hearing aids

These comprise a titanium screw abutment and an external hearing aid processor. Titanium screws can be implanted into bone and become firmly anchored. This enables them to have a hearing aid attached and allow sound to be transmitted to the cochlea via bone conduction. Useful in patients with atresia of the ear canal, or in those who cannot have conventional aids, e.g. continuous ear discharge with the conventional occlusive aids.

Cochlear implants

When profound hearing loss exists which cannot be adequately amplified, a cochlear implant can provide some help. Normal cochlear structure is essential. A multichannel electrode is inserted into the cochlea surgically. It directly stimulates the cochlea when electrical signals are applied. Each channel corresponds to a different frequency. The electrode is attached to an external auditory processor through the skin via a magnetic coupler. Sound is collected and processed and fed to the channels on the electrode. Some sound is perceived to enable enhanced lip reading or just to give some environmental feedback. Patients may have excellent hearing and can even conduct conversations over the telephone.

Brainstem auditory implants

This is the only option for the profoundly deaf person without a normal functioning cochlea. Electrodes are placed on the auditory pathway to stimulate the cochlear nucleus directly. Results are not as good as cochlear implantation but some sound is perceived.

Skull base

Overview

The skull base is a specialized area of clinical work. The ENT surgeon is actively involved in this area, often as part of a team which includes a neurosurgeon or plastic surgeon.

Access to these difficult areas has been increased with the development of image guidance systems.

Acoustic neuroma

Acoustic neuroma is a benign, slow-growing tumour. It is more correctly called a 'vestibular Schwannoma', because of its origin on the vestibular nerve. Postmortem data shows that it is underdiagnosed. An acoustic neuroma may be discovered serendipitously on an MRI scan for another condition.

Acoustic neuromas account for 6% of all intracranial neoplasms, the majority of which are sporadic (95%). Some 5% are genetic—part of the inherited condition of NF2 (Neurofibromatosis Type 2) a chromosome 22 abnormality.

Presentation

The patient may experience some of the following:
- Sudden SNHL or progressive high-frequency SNHL
- Vertiginous episodes—but these are rare as the patient unknowingly compensates
- Symptoms of raised intracranial pressure—such as headache or visual disturbance
- Brainstem compression—ataxia is a late symptom of this

Investigations

- PTA
- MRI scan with gadolinium contrast
- Full otoneurological exam, paying particular attention to:
  - Hitselberger's sign—postauricular numbness due to facial nerve compression
  - reduced corneal reflex
  - Unterburger's test positive—patient marches on the spot with the eyes closed. A positive test is a rotation to one side or the other

Management

Management options balance the risk of hearing loss, facial nerve palsy, and surgical morbidity. There are several possibilities:
- Watchful waiting—with serial MRI scans for slow-growing tumours
- Surgical excision via:
  - retrosigmoid approach—likely to preserve the hearing
  - translabyrinthine approach—destroys the hearing but is an easier approach. It is useful if there is little hearing to preserve
  - middle fossa approach—is technically challenging as it involves opening the middle fossa. No driving for one year (UK) due to the risk of seizures
  - intracapsular removal—used in elderly or infirm patients who need brainstem decompression rather than total tumour removal
- Stereotactic radiosurgery—this multiplanar radiotherapy is useful in the treatment of small tumours, as it avoids surgery.

Complications
- Any procedure which involves a craniotomy carries a 1% risk of death
- Facial nerve palsy
- Total hearing loss

Differential diagnosis of cerebellopontine angle (CPA) tumour

- Acoustic neuroma 80%
- Meningioma
- Epidermoid cyst
- Cholesterol granuloma
- Arachnoid cyst
- Posterior cerebellar artery (PCA) aneurysm

Nasopharyngeal carcinoma

There are two distinct types of this cancer of the back of the nose:
- Undifferentiated non-keratinizing SCC—this is more common in people from southern China and Chinese people from Hong Kong. It is associated with the Epstein–Bar virus (EBV).
- Differentiated keratinizing SCC—this has similar at-risk groups to the majority of head and neck cancers.

Presentation
- Epistaxis 77%
- Nasal obstruction
- Headaches 73%
- Lymph node metastasis 60%
- Middle ear effusion
- Extensive tumours can involve the skull base and cause cranial nerve palsies

Examination
Full endoscopic evaluation including visualization of the larynx with the flexible nasendoscope. Cranial nerve examination (25% involved at presentation)

Investigations
Patients will require a CT/MRI scan.

Important

Every patient presenting with a unilateral middle ear effusion must have their postnasal space visualized to exclude a nasopharyngeal carcinoma.

Treatment
- Radiotherapy is given for all stages. Neck dissection may be necessary if there are extensive lymph node metastases.

Anatomical subdivisions of nasopharynx
- Posterior superior wall—skull base to the level of the hard palate
- Lateral wall—eustachian tube opening (ETO) and the fossa of Rosenmüller
- Inferior wall—superior surface of soft palate

T stage of nasopharyngeal carcinoma
- **T1**—limited to 1 subsite
- **T2**—involvement of more than 1 subsite
- **T3**—invasion of oral cavity/oropharynx
- **T4**—invasion of skull base/cranial nerve involvement

Juvenile nasal angiofibroma (JNA)

This is a rare tumour almost exclusively seen in males. Females with JNA should have genetic investigation.

Usually presents in the second decade of life. Rarely >25 years.

It originates from the sphenopalatine foramen, is locally invasive but not malignant, and is a combination of fibrous tissue with endothelial spaces in vascular tissue.

Symptoms
- Nasal obstruction 80%
- Recurrent epistaxis 50–60%
- Headache 25%
- Facial swelling 5%

Signs
- Nasal mass
- Orbital mass
- Proptosis

Investigations
- Clinical examination with endoscope
- CT scan and MRI
- Angiography
- Do *not* biopsy for fear of life-threatening haemorrhage

Management
The treatment is surgical removal, with preoperative embolization to reduce the blood loss during the operation. There are several ways to gain access to the area, but the most common is via the face using a 'midfacial degloving' procedure.

Radiotherapy can be used.

Fisch classification of JNA
Stage I—tumours limited to nasal cavity, nasopharynx with no bony destruction

Stage II—tumours invading the pterygomaxillary fossa or paranasal sinuses with bony destruction

Stage III—tumours invading infratemporal fossa, orbit, and/or parasellar region remaining lateral to cavernous sinus

Stage IV—tumours invading cavernous sinus, optic chiasmal region, and/or pituitary fossa

Sinonasal malignancy

This term describes a diverse group of malignant tumours affecting the nose and sinus system. Squamous cell carcinoma (SCC) accounts for 70% of sinonasal malignancy, adenocarcinoma 10%, and adenoid cystic carcinoma 10%.

Nickel workers are at risk of developing SCC, woodworkers are at risk of adenocarcinoma. This is often delayed up to 20 years after exposure.

The prognosis is poor with less than a 50% 5-year survival rate.

Common sites for sinonasal malignancy

- Maxillary sinus
- Nasal cavity
- Ethmoid sinus

Presentation

Some or all of the following features may be seen:

- Nasal obstruction
- Epistaxis
- Sinusitis
- Maxillary symptoms:
  - loose teeth
  - pain/ulceration of palate
  - cheek swelling
- Ethmoid symptoms:
  - unilateral obstruction
  - diplopia
  - headache

Investigations

- CT and/or MRI
- Endoscopy and biopsy
- Fine needle aspiration (FNA) if cervical metastases

Treatment

Surgical resection and/or radiotherapy may be required. Treatment decisions should be made in a head and neck MDT meeting, taking into account the histological type and grade of tumour, the staging, as well as the patient's medical status and wishes.

The nose and sinuses

Structure and function of the nose

Structure

The structure of the nose is made up of four parts:

- The surface anatomy—📖 see Fig. 9.1.
- The nasal skeleton—composed of the two nasal bones, the paired upper lateral and lower lateral cartilages and the nasal septum, covered in subcutaneous tissue and skin (Figs 9.2–9.4).
- The internal anatomy—includes the septum of the nose which forms the medial wall of the paired nasal cavities. The turbinates, also called conchae (the Latin term for scroll, which describes their appearance neatly) are attached to the lateral wall.
- The osteomeatal complex—a key functional area of the nose. Understanding its anatomy is essential in understanding the aetiology of sinus disease.

Knowing the anatomical terms for parts of the nose helps you to describe the site of lesions accurately, and to document the findings of examinations accurately.

Function

The nose is the main route for inspired air, and its structure is related to this function. As the air passes over the large surface area of the turbinates, the inspired gases are warmed and humidified. Mucus on the mucosa of the nose removes large dust particles from the air as it is breathed in (as anyone who has blown their nose after a trip on the London underground knows!).

The voice resonates in the sinuses and nose and this provides character to the speech. Patients with very obstructed nasal passages have what is often described as a 'hyponasal' quality to their speech.

Pneumatization of the sinuses are air-filled spaces, which reduces the weight of the skull.

The specialized neuroepithelium in the roof of the nose is the sire of olfactory sensation.

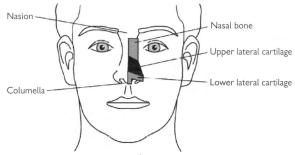

Fig. 9.1 Diagram of the surface landmarks of the nose.

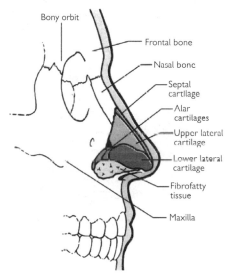

Fig. 9.2 Diagram of the nasal skeleton.

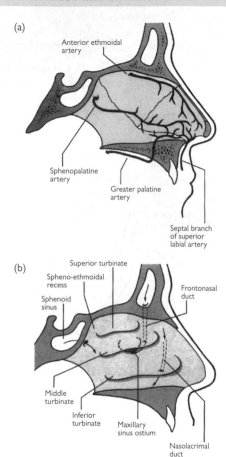

Fig. 9.3 Diagram of the internal structure of the nose.

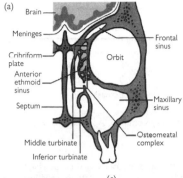

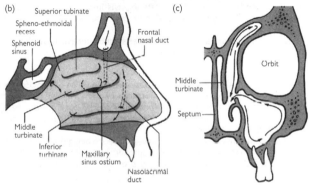

Fig. 9.4 The osteomeatal complex.

Rhinitis

Rhinitis is an inflammation of the nasal lining. Rhinitis may be diagnosed if a patient has two out of the three symptoms for more than 1h every day for over 2 weeks.

Symptoms
- Blocked nose
- Running nose—including postnasal drip
- Sneezing

This condition is very common. Approximately one in six adults suffers from rhinitis.

Causes

There are a multitude of factors which cause rhinitis. However, since it may be caused by several different factors, it is important to treat each different cause. The symptoms of rhinitis may also be part of systemic disease (Table 9.1).

The commonest forms of rhinitis are allergic and infective. Classification of the disease and its rarer forms are shown in Table 9.1.

History

It is important to take a full history to determine the cause of rhinitis. This includes asking the patient about any history of atopy or asthma, and any seasonal variation in the symptoms. Documenting the main symptoms—blockage, running, and sneezing—and noting which one is predominant will help in treatment selection.

The patient should be asked what medications are being used and about their smoking history—almost every smoker has a degree of rhinitis. The patient should be asked about any previous treatment for rhinitis, including its duration and effectiveness.

Investigations
- Anterior rhinoscopy—looking for enlarged turbinates (a blue tinge often indicates an allergic rhinitis) or nasal polyps.
- Nasal endoscopy—examining the middle meatus for mucus or polyps.
- Skin prick allergy tests—tiny amounts of test substances are placed on the skin and a pin prick is made—a positive result leads to a small raised, red, itchy patch.
- RAST tests—a blood test which indicates if patients are allergic to a range of test substances.
- Peak flow—many patients with rhinitis also have asthma—their peak flow test may be reduced.

Types of rhinitis

Table 9.1 Types of rhinitis

Common			Rare
Allergic	Infective	Other	Part of systemic disease
Seasonal	Acute	Idiopathic	Primary mucus defect
Perennial	Chronic	NARES (non-allergic	Cystic fibrosis
Occupational		rhinitis with eosinophilia)	Young's disease
		Drug-induced	Primary ciliary dyskinesia
		beta-blockers	Kartagener's syndrome
		Oral contraceptives	Immunological
		Aspirin	SLE
		NSAIDs	Rheumatoid arthritis
		Local decongestants	AIDS
		Autonomic	Antibody deficiency
		Atrophic	Granulomatous disease
		Neoplastic	Wegener's/sarcoidosis
			Hormonal
			Hypothyroidism
			Pregnancy
			Old man's drip

Medical treatment of rhinitis

The treatment of rhinitis is related to the underlying aetiology of the condition. Medical treatment is given if the patient feels their symptoms are bad enough.

Allergen avoidance

If the patient's rhinitis is caused by an allergy, skin prick testing can identify the allergens to be avoided. It gives a visual feedback to the patient to confirm the diagnosis. Following a positive skin prick test, the patient can be given allergen avoidance information both verbally and on information sheets.

Pharmacological treatments

Each of the different medications has different effects on symptoms (Table 9.2).

- **Steroids**—should ideally be delivered topically to the nasal mucosa using sprays or drops.
- **Oral steroids**—can be very effective but their systemic effects limit their long-term use. A short course can be ideal for an important summer event such as an exam or a wedding, e.g. prednisolone PO od 0.5mg/kg for 1 week.
- **Antihistamines**—non-sedating antihistamines are effective against sneezing, itching, and watery rhinorrhoea, e.g. cetirizine 10mg od PO. Used systemically they can be effective for other atopic problems such as watery eyes. They are not useful for symptoms of blockage.
- **Nasal decongestants**—are only useful in the short term at the start of other therapy or when flying, since prolonged use can produce the intractable rhinorrhoea of rhinitis medicamentosa. For example, oxymetazoline 0.5% 2 drops bd into both nostrils for 2 weeks.
- **Ipratropium bromide**—is an intranasal preparation and is effective for watery vasomotor-type rhinitis, e.g. ipratropium bromide 0.03% 2 sprays qds into both nostrils.
- **Sodium cromoglicate**—is a mast cell stabilizer and is useful for allergic rhinitis. Sodium cromoglicate 4% 2 sprays each nostril qds.

Tabel 9.2 Effects of various drugs on rhinitis

	Sneezing	Discharge	Blockage	Anosmia
Cromoglicate	++	+	+	–
Decongestant	–	–	+++	–
Antihistamine	+++	++	±	–
Ipratropium	–	++	–	–
Topical steroids	+++	++	++	+
Oral steroids	++	++	+++	++

Surgical treatment of rhinitis

The role of surgery is limited in the treatment of rhinitis. Surgery to improve nasal function may be a useful adjunct to other treatments.

Even if a surgically correctable problem is found it is worth a trial of medical therapy alone in the first instance. There is often a high rate of symptom resolution.

It is worth obtaining a CT scan of the paranasal sinuses if surgery is considered to review the need for sinus surgery.

Turbinate reduction

The turbinates often hypertrophy in all types of rhinitis but particularly in allergic rhinitis. Their hypertrophy often obstructs the airway to such a degree that it is impossible to deliver topical medication. Reduction can be achieved by several means:

• Surface linear cautery—burning the surface
• Submucous diathermy—burning under the surface
• Cryotherapy—freezing
• Outfracture— pushing out of the airway
• Submucosal conchopexy—changing the shape of the turbinate
• Trimming or cutting the turbinate

These techniques are effective in improving the airway for 18 months, but additional medical therapy is needed to prevent recurrence of the hypertrophied mucosa. The technique of trimming has a better long-term result, but has the potential for severe postoperative haemorrhage. Surgeons undertaking this type of surgery are known as turbinate terrorists!

Septal surgery

A deviated septum may need to be corrected to improve nasal function and help medication delivery.

Functional endoscopic sinus surgery

This surgery is aimed at the osteomeatal complex—it aims to remove blockage in the critical area and restore the normal function and drainage of the sinuses. It could benefit patients with sinusitis who do not respond to medical treatments.

Sinusitis

Sinusitis is a common inflammation of the sinuses. It is now regarded as a continuation of the spectrum of rhinitis.

The work of Messerklinger has shown that effective sinus drainage occurs through the area known as the osteomeatal complex (□ see Fig. 9.4). Obstruction in this area due to anatomical or mucosal problems impairs sinus drainage and leads to obstructed outflow. This can occur as an acute phenomenon (□ see 'Acute sinusitis', p. 170) or as a chronic condition (□ see 'Chronic sinusitis', p. 172).

Other theories of sinusitis are especially relevant to surgical failures (10–30%) where the sinus outflow tracts are open and the patient clinically still has mucopurulent secretions coming from their sinuses.

Fungal sinusitis

Fungi can be inhaled into the sinus tracts and can promote a prolonged chronic inflammation that causes sinus symptoms. This is mediated by an IgE response. Fungi can be isolated from the sinuses in almost 100% of patients, so the causality is doubted.

Biofilm production

Free-floating organisms form a biofilm by becoming anchored to a mucosal surface. The organisms then become more organized and progressively more difficult to remove from the surface. This facilitates further organism attachment. The expanding biofilm may destroy cilia and goblet cells of the normal sinus mucosa. This can lead to sinusitis and antibiotic resistance. Some studies have shown a very high percentage of biofilms in patients with sinusitis.

Superantigens

Colonization by *Staphylococcal aureus* with the production of enterotoxin can generate a potent immune response. These are known as 'superantigens'. This leads to activation of the immune cascade and can lead to the development of chronic sinusitis. IgE antibodies to *S. aureus* enterotoxin have been isolated in 50–90% of patients with nasal polyposis.

Acute sinusitis

It is thought that everyone will suffer from an episode of sinusitis at some time in their life. It is caused by an acute bacterial infection which often develops after a preceding viral illness, such as a cold.

Signs and symptoms
- Preceding URTI
- Nasal obstruction
- Severe facial pain over the sinuses, particularly the maxillae/cheeks
- Pain, which is worse on bending down or coughing

A swelling on the face is usually caused by a dental abscess rather than by sinus disease. Tenderness over the sinuses is an overemphasized sign.

Investigations
- Anterior rhinoscopy—to examine the inside of the nose
- Nasal endoscopy—often shows the presence of pus in the middle meatus or oedematous mucosa

Treatment
In previously healthy adults, medication alone is usually effective:
- Antibiotics may be given—co-amoxiclav 625mg PO tds 1/52
- Decongestant—xylometazoline 0.1% drops 2 drops tds 1/52
- Anti-inflammatory betamethasone drops—2 drops bd into both nostrils

If sinus symptoms do not resolve, consider sinus washout or endoscopic sinus surgery after CT to confirm the diagnosis.

In immunocompromised patients, consider a sinus washout to obtain microbiology for more effective antimicrobial treatment. Also, seek advice from local microbiologists for other appropriate therapy.

> **Tip**: A pledget soaked in 5% cocaine solution placed in the middle meatus under endoscopic guidance may relieve the obstructed osteo-meatal complex due to its intense vasoconstriction.

Recurrent acute sinusitis

Patients presenting with a history of recurrent sinusitis are often difficult to diagnose. This is because in the absence of an acute infection there may be no abnormal physical signs. Even CT scans may be entirely normal.

If the history is good, functional endoscopic sinus surgery (FESS) is appropriate if the number of episodes of infection is sufficient to cause disruption to the person's lifestyle.

To avoid misdiagnosis, patients can be given an open appointment to turn up when their symptoms are severe. Endoscopic examination at this time may reveal pus in the middle meatus. When a patient is symptomatic a CT scan can also be helpful, but this depends on a co-operative radiology department who will allow rapid access.

◑ Differential diagnosis of sinusitis

- Migraine—typical or non-classical migraine symptoms may mimic sinus symptoms
- Dental problems—abscess or temporomandibular joint disorders
- Trigeminal neuralgia
- Neuralgias of uncertain origin
- Atypical facial pain

Remember that the CT paranasal sinus scan may be normal unless the patient is symptomatic.

Beware of operating on patients where there is no good evidence of sinus disease on a CT scan or on endoscopic examination—the results of surgery in this group are disappointing.

Chronic sinusitis

Chronic sinusitis is an inflammation of the sinuses lasting more than 6 weeks. Diagnosing chronic sinusitis, like diagnosing acute sinusitis, may be difficult, as it may be mimicked by other causes of facial pain.

Signs and symptoms
- Pressure in the face—which gets worse on bending over
- Pain when flying—in particular when descending
- A feeling of nasal obstruction
- Rhinitis—runny or blocked nose and sneezing

Investigations
- Nasal examination—to check the patency of the airway
- Anterior rhinoscopy—to examine the septum and nasal cavity
- Posterior rhinoscopy with rigid endoscope—to examine the middle meatus and look for nasal polyps

Treatment
Some 80% of patients respond to medical therapy. This will involve one or more of the following medications for at least 3 months:
- Intranasal steroid—mild inflammation/oedema in the nose, e.g. fluticasone two sprays od into both nostrils. For gross oedema a higher concentration of steroids is needed—for example betamethasone drops, 2 drops bd into both nostrils.
- Oral antihistamine—e.g. cetirizine hydrochloride 10mg od PO.

If medical treatment fails, the following treatments may be considered:
- A CT scan—to provide a surgical road map
- FESS—extent dictated by disease process at surgery
- Septoplasty—may be necessary in addition to the above

Surgery for chronic rhinosinusitis

Indications
- Failed medical therapy
- Surgically treatable sinus disease

Methods
FESS (functional endoscopic sinus surgery)
Most sinus surgery is now carried out with the use of Hopkins rod endoscopes and based on the original theories of Messerklinger. Obstruction at the osteomeatal complex is relieved by surgically enlarging the common drainage pathway of the sinuses. Thus it is functional surgery—opening up the natural drainage pathways.

The extent of the sinus surgery depends on the distribution of disease and the abilities of the surgeon. A progressive approach would be to carry out the following procedures:
- Uncinectomy
- Middle meatal antrostomy
- Opening of the bulla ethmoidalis
- Anterior and posterior ethmoidectomies
- Sphenoidotomies
- Opening of the frontal recess and ensuring drainage of the frontal sinuses

Complications
Rare—orbital ecchymosis, orbital haemorrhage, CSF leak, orbital damage including optic nerve injury.

Extended procedures
The following are often used to treat extensive polypoid disease or recurrent disease:
Canine fossa puncture—here a sublabial incision enables access to the front wall of the maxillary sinus. A trocar passed through the bone of the maxilla enables passage of instruments to access the front inner face of the maxillary sinus. The procedure can lead to numbness of the upper lip and cheek.
Modified Lothrop procedure—this is performed for the treatment of persistent frontal sinusitis and usually reserved for revision cases. Image-guided surgery equipment is used and the frontal recess is widened anteriorly in a U-shape fashion, including removal of the top part of the septum. This provides drainage of the frontal sinuses.
Balloon sinuplasty—is a new treatment which uses the principles of Messerklinger's theories. A balloon is passed into the sinus to be treated using a guidewire technique. This is particularly useful for the frontal sinus. The balloon is then inflated to widen the sinus outflow tract. Irrigation catheters can then be placed into the sinus for delivery of topical steroids or antibiotics. However, the technique does not treat the mucosal inflammation in the ethmoidal sinuses. Balloon techniques can dilate obstructed frontal, maxillary, and sphenoid sinuses.

Ethmoidal implants, e.g. Stratos™—a patented drug delivery system for the ethmoid has been developed. This implant is inserted under radiological control and positioned in the anterior and posterior ethmoid anterior to the face of the sphenoid sinus. It can be filled with long-acting steroid (triamcinolone) which is released over a period of 30 days.

Complications of sinusitis

Mucociliary damage

Long-standing or chronic sinusitis can lead to mucociliary failure. This means that the sinus cannot drain properly, even if it is anatomically ventilated. Cigarette smoke will also paralyse cilia action, so smoking should be avoided by those with sinusitis.

Orbital complications

An unresolved episode of acute ethmoid or pansinusitis may lead to orbital complications, as shown in Figs 9.5 and 9.6. Infection under pressure in the ethmoid sinuses can traverse the thin bony plate of the medial orbital wall. This can lead to oedema formation and abscess formation. The management of this problem is dealt with in the Emergencies section of this book (see 'Periorbital cellulitis', p. 380). The Chandler classification of orbital complications is shown in Fig. 9.5.

Intracranial complications

Infection under pressure in the frontal sinus can lead to stasis of blood in the diploeic veins which traverse the skull. Infection can travel back through the posterior table of the frontal sinus into the cranial cavity. This can lead to meningeal irritation, cerebral oedema, and frontal lobe abscess formation.

Pott's puffy tumour

Ongoing frontal sinusitis can lead to osteomyelitis of the frontal bone. A soft boggy swelling then appears on the skin of the forehead. It was given this colourful name by Percival Pott.

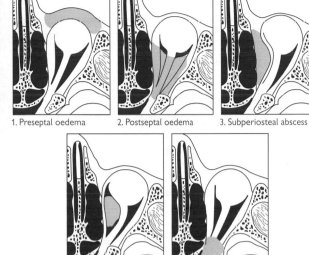

1. Preseptal oedema   2. Postseptal oedema   3. Subperiosteal abscess

4. Interconal abscess   5. Cavernous sinus
                            involvement

Fig. 9.5 Chandler classification of orbital complications.

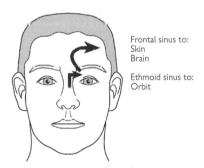

Frontal sinus to:
Skin
Brain

Ethmoid sinus to:
Orbit

Fig. 9.6 Pathways of spread for intracranial complications.

Nasal polyps

Simple nasal polyps are part of the spectrum of rhinosinusitis as the lining of the nose becomes inflamed and thicker. These polyps are oedematous sinus mucosa, which prolapse to fill the nasal cavity to a variable extent. They are common, and their cause is unknown.

Signs and symptoms
- Variable symptoms—with the season or with URTI
- Rhinitis—blocked or runny nose and sneezing
- Sinusitis—due to osteomeatal obstruction
- Nasal obstruction
- Appearance of the polyps at the anterior nares

Investigations
- Anterior rhinoscopy—inferior turbinates are often incorrectly diagnosed as polyps, a rhinoscopy can help avoid this misdiagnosis (Fig. 9.7)
- Nasal endoscopy—examination of the nose with an endoscope
- Polyp size—can be graded (Fig. 9.8)

Treatment
- **For small nasal polyps**—give topical steroids, e.g. betamethasone drops: 2 drops bd for 2 weeks, followed by fluticasone 2 sprays od into both nostrils for 3 months
- **For large nasal polyps**—give oral steroids 30mg od for 1 week, followed by fluticasone 2 sprays bd for 3 months

If medical treatment fails, the following should be considered:
- Surgical removal for obstructive polyps—if the patient is sufficiently symptomatic
- A CT scan to provide a road map prior to more advanced surgery
- FESS—using a microdebrider for atraumatic polypectomy
- Postoperative intranasal steroids to prevent recurrence

Samter's triad associated polyp
This is the association of:
- Aspirin sensitivity—making patients wheezy when they take aspirin
- Late-onset asthma
- Nasal polyps
- It is caused by a defect in leukotriene metabolism. Polyps in this condition are florid and recur frequently

Treatment
- Diet—refer patient to a dietician for advice on a low salicylate diet. This is very bland and difficult to maintain.
- Intranasal steroids—patients often elect to use betamethasone drops long term despite their risk of systemic side effects.
- Repeat surgery as for nasal polyps above—the microdebrider is the atraumatic instrument of choice.
- Leukotriene antagonists, e.g. montelukast—aim to reduce polyps, results may vary.

Danger signs

A unilateral polyp must be regarded as a malignancy until proven otherwise by a biopsy.

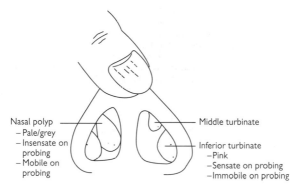

Nasal polyp
– Pale/grey
– Insensate on probing
– Mobile on probing

Middle turbinate

Inferior turbinate
– Pink
– Sensate on probing
– Immobile on probing

Fig. 9.7 Diagram of nasal polyp showing features compared with inferior turbinate.

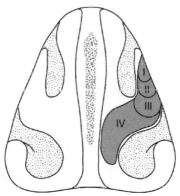

Fig. 9.8 Polyp size can be graded.

Unusual nasal polyps

Antrochoanal polyps

These originate from the maxillary sinus and often present as a unilateral pendulous mass in the nasopharynx (Fig. 9.9). The uncinate process directs the polyp posteriorly as it emerges from the maxillary sinus. They are uncommon and their cause is not known.

Macroscopically, the polyp is formed from a nasal component which is similar in appearance to a common nasal polyp.

The maxillary antral component is a thin fluid-filled cyst. A small fibrous band joins the two components as it passes out through the expanded sinus otium.

Treatment

- CT scan—to confirm the diagnosis.
- Endoscopic removal of the polyps—from its point of attachment in the maxillary sinus.
- Caldwell–Luc approach for recurrent problem—an open sinus operation accessing the sinus via a cut in the mouth under the top lip.

Childhood polyps

Polyps presenting in childhood are very unusual. They are usually associated with an underlying mucociliary abnormality such as cystic fibrosis or primary ciliary dyskinesia syndrome.

Investigations

- Consider a sweat test—the diagnostic test for cystic fibrosis
- Histology—send samples for histology to exclude a tumour
- Fresh sample of nasal lining—for special tests of ciliary function
- Sample for electron microscopy—to check ciliary structure

Treatments

- Medical treatment with steroids, e.g. prednisolone 1mg/kg for 1 week
- Surgical removal

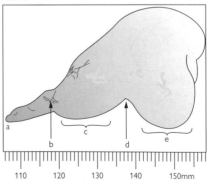

Fig. 9.9 An antrochoanal polyp and its anatomical relations. a = maxillary sinus attachment; b = maxillary ostium; c = osteomeatal complex; d = posterior choana; e = nasopharynx.

Septal problems

The nasal septum provides an important mechanical support for the external nasal skeleton.

Problems with the nasal septum can lead to both a cosmetic and functional disturbance of the nose. The nose may look bent to one side and/or the nasal airway may be restricted.

Septal deviation

The causes of septal deviation can be either congenital or traumatic. A traumatic septal deviation could be the result of a broken nose. Congenital septal deviation can occur after birth trauma to the nose, or the differential growth of the nasal septum compared to the rest of the skull.

Almost all nasal septae are deviated to some extent. Most people do not experience any problems, but some find their airway has become restricted.

Acoustic rhinomanometry and computer flow modelling has shown that deviations at the area of the nasal valve cause most functional impairment to airflow. This area is situated about 1cm posterior to the nares. It is bounded superiorly by the overlap of the upper and lower lateral cartilages. Laterally is the origin of the anterior part of the inferior turbinate; inferiorly, the floor of the nose; and medially, the nasal septum. Changes in the relative position of any of these structures causes a change in the area of the nasal valve.

Investigations
- Anterior rhinoscopy—to exclude other problems, e.g. rhinitis
- Cottle's test—to exclude alar collapse
- Nasendoscopy—to exclude sinusitis

Treatment
- Medical—3-month trial of an intranasal steroid, e.g. betamethasone nasal spray 2 drops bd into both nostrils.
- Surgical—septoplasty or a submucous resection (SMR) is an operation on the nasal septum to improve nasal airflow.

Septal perforation

There are several reasons why a patient's septum may be perforated. These include:

- Trauma or accident
- Postseptal surgery
- Nose picking
- Granulomatous disease—must be excluded before treating perforation (📖 see 'Granulomatous conditions', p. 183).
- Wegener's
- Sarcoidosis
- TB
- Syphilis
- Cocaine addiction

Signs and symptoms

- Whistling—if there is a small anterior perforation
- Bleeding from the nose
- Crusting of the nose at the site of the perforation

Treatment

- Patient applies a lump of petroleum jelly, on the end of their little finger, twice daily to the edge of the perforation.
- Epistaxis treated using silver nitrate cautery. Often occurs from the posterior edge of the perforation.
- Septal button—this is a plastic prosthesis fitted into the hole in the septum. Only half of patients find it tolerable and continue using it long term.
- Surgical septal repair—the results of surgery are variable even in experienced hands.

Granulomatous conditions

These are an uncommon group of diseases which are classified together because of their histological appearance—all of which form granulomas. These conditions include:

- Wegener's granulomatosis—is a multisystem disease characterized by perivascular granuloma formation, which most often affects the respiratory system and the kidneys.
- Sarcoidosis—its cause is unknown.
- Syphilis—a sexually transmitted disease which can affect the nose.

Signs and symptoms

- The patient may present with systemic symptoms, e.g. sarcoid with chest problems.
- Patients may have isolated nasal symptoms, such as septal perforation (posterior in syphilis) or crusting on the nasal septum.

Investigations

- FBC
- U+Es
- ESR
- Syphilis serology
- ANCA
- CXR
- Nasal biopsy

Treatment

Involve the medical team who deal with the condition in hospital, such as the chest or renal teams. They can assess the patient for signs of systemic disease.

Further medical treatment is managed by the appropriate medical team, often with immunosuppressants.

Sinonasal malignancy

Sinonasal malignancy is not a common condition.
  The common types of malignancy are:
- Squamous cell carcinoma
- Malignant melanoma
- Adenocarcinoma of the ethmoid
- Olfactory neuroblastoma

Symptoms
- Nasal polyp with obstruction
- Epistaxis
- Cacosmia = unpleasant smell from the nose experienced by patients
- Cranial nerve palsies
- Proptosis

Assessment
- Nasal endoscopy
- CT scan
- MRI scan—helps to detect intracranial spread
- Angiography—for assessment and possible embolization prior to surgical resection

Treatment
Following tumour staging a treatment plan is formulated by the MDT in the skull base clinic. The team involves ENT, neurosurgery, and plastic surgeons.
  Craniofacial resection is standard care.
  Endoscopic combined resection is becoming more widespread.

The mouth, tonsils, and adenoids

Anatomy

The nose and throat

The nose and throat can be divided into the following anatomical areas (Fig. 10.1):

- **Oral cavity**—extends from the lips to the anterior pillar of the tonsil.
- **Oropharynx**—extends from the anterior pillar to the posterior pharyngeal wall. It contains the tonsils and the base of the tongue.
- **Nasopharynx**—located above the level of the palate and contains the adenoids. The Eustachian tubes open into it laterally and it communicates with the nasal cavity anteriorly.

The tongue

The anterior third and posterior two-thirds of the tongue have different embryological origins, and different nerve supplies.

- **Motor supply** to the tongue is via the hypoglossal nerve.
- **Sensation** to the anterior two-thirds of the tongue is via the lingual nerve. The posterior third is supplied by the glossopharyngeal nerve.
- **Taste** fibres pass with the facial nerve to the middle ear. From here they separate—as the chorda tympani—and pass forwards. As they exit the middle ear they merge with the mandibular division of the trigeminal nerve to eventually run with the lingual nerve.

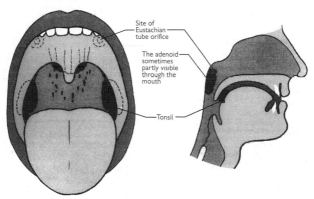

Fig. 10.1 Oral cavity AP and oropharynx/nasopharynx lateral.

Oral ulcers—benign

Traumatic ulcers

Acute traumatic ulcers are common, they heal quickly, and patients rarely seek any medical attention. Chronic traumatic ulcers are seen more often. These can arise from ill-fitting dentures, sharp or rotten teeth. They usually occur on the lateral aspect of the tongue, or on the inside of the cheek. The only treatment required is a dental review or a refitting of the denture.

Aphthous ulcers

These are the common mouth ulcers that most people will suffer from at some time in their lives. They are small and painful and usually appear in crops. They most often affect the lateral border or the tip of the tongue, but they may occur anywhere in the oral cavity. It is unclear what causes them, but hormonal changes, poor oral hygiene, trauma, poor diet, and stress have all been suggested as factors. Usually, these ulcers present little more than a minor irritation for 24–48 hours. However, occasionally they are severe and recurrent. Treatment in this case should consist of simple analgesia, local anaesthetic gels, or steroid pastels. Rarely, a single giant aphthous ulcer may develop. This can look alarming or may even appear malignant. In this case, a biopsy may be necessary.

Infective ulcers

Herpes simplex may cause mouth ulcers which look similar to aphthous ulcers. However, the patient will often have additional symptoms of mild pyrexia and malaise. Aciclovir is effective if given in the early stages. Herpes zoster may affect the oral cavity, but is usually seen in immuno-compromised and debilitated patients.

The 'snail track' ulcers of syphilis are rarely seen. Oral ulceration along with candidiasis, tonsillitis, Kaposi's sarcoma, and hairy leukoplakia are all features of AIDS infection.

Dietary and blood disorders

Deficiencies in iron, folate, and vitamin B_{12} can cause oral ulceration, since these agents are required for normal mucosal development. Mouth ulcers also occur as a result of leukaemia, polycythaemia, and agranulocytosis. Signs of scurvy and pellagra include a sore mouth and ulceration.

Torus palatinus

This is a benign osteoma on the hard palate. Its surface may become ulcerated, usually as a result of trauma from an overlying denture. In this case the lesion may look and feel malignant. These lesions need only be removed if they interfere with the fitting of a dental plate.

Oral ulcers—malignant

Squamous cell carcinoma

This is the commonest malignant lesion found in the mouth. Risk factors include smoking, drinking alcohol (in particular spirits), chewing betel nuts, and having sharp teeth.

Symptoms and signs

It usually starts as an ulcer, often on the lateral border of the tongue, the floor of the mouth, or the gum. These ulcers progress and are painful, often with referred pain to the ear. Malignant ulcers of the tongue may be superficial or deeply infiltrating, but in either case they usually feel hard.

Investigations

More information can usually be gathered from palpation than from inspection. It is vital to adequately examine the neck for lymph node metastasis, paying particular attention to the submandibular and submental triangles as well as those nodes deep to the sternomastoid running along the internal jugular vein. SCC of the oral cavity will most commonly metastasize to the nodes in levels 1, 2, and 3 (📖 see 'Lymph node levels', p. 262). An MRI scan or a spiral CT scan is most often employed to assess the neck. In skilled hands, ultrasound-guided FNA is a highly sensitive and specific tool in assessing the neck.

Management

Any ulcer that fails to heal within two weeks should be biopsied to exclude malignancy. Many patients who develop oral cavity SCC have widespread mucosal field change as a result of their smoking and drinking. They are at high risk of developing another upper aerodigestive tract cancer at the same time or at some time in the future. All patients presenting with SCC should have a panendoscopy under GA to exclude any additional primary tumour. The panendoscopy will also allow proper assessment of the primary tumour.

Treatment

Options include both external beam and interstitial radiotherapy as well as surgical en-bloc resection of all the affected hard and soft tissues. The surgically created defect will require reconstruction to produce an acceptable functional and cosmetic result for the patient.

White patches in the mouth

There are many possible causes of white patches in the mouth. These include:

Candida

Candida tends to occur in debilitated and immunocompromised patients. White specks coalesce to form patches, or a white membrane, which when lifted reveals a red raw mucosal surface. It sometimes occurs on the soft palate and can complicate the use of steroid inhalers in asthma patients. Candida is usually diagnosed by looking at it, but if any doubt remains, scrapings of the lesion should be taken and sent for microbiological examination.

Leukoplakia

Any white patch in the mouth can be called leukoplakia, but it usually refers to hyperkeratosis of the oral mucosa. This happens to patients who share the same risk factors as those who develop SCC: smoking, alcohol, strong spices, and prolonged irritation from sharp teeth or poorly fitting false teeth. This lesion is premalignant and 3% will undergo malignant change within five years of diagnosis. A biopsy and regular reviews are essential. A particular form of leukoplakia known as 'hairy leukoplakia' occurs in AIDS patients; the condition is so named because of its histological appearance.

Lichen planus

This condition usually occurs on the inside of the cheek and has a white lace-like appearance. It may be extremely painful but usually responds to topical steroid preparations. The aetiology remains unclear.

Mucus retention cysts

These usually form a smooth, pale, round swelling which may occur anywhere in the oral cavity, base of the tongue, or the tonsils. These swellings arise from a blockage in one of the many mucous glands found throughout the upper aerodigestive tract mucosa. Reassurance is usually all that is required. If there is any diagnostic uncertainty, or if they become large enough to cause symptoms as a result of their size, then excision/ marsupialization may be required.

Miscellaneous mouth conditions

Geographic tongue
This is a common condition where depapillation of the tongue surface occurs as red patches with a white border. The sites vary and seem to move around the tongue. The cause is unknown but it often runs in families. Reassurance is the only treatment required.

Angioedema
This allergic reaction causes generalized swelling of the tongue. Seafood, peanuts, and drugs such as lisinopril can all have this effect. The swelling may progress rapidly and obstruct the patient's airway. Medical treatment consists of intravenous steroids, piriton, and nebulized adrenaline. The airway may need to be secured either by endotracheal intubation or tracheostomy.

Median rhomboid glossitis
This appears as a raised smooth patch in the centre of the dorsum of the tongue. It has been linked with reflux and candida infection. In most cases simple reassurance is all that is required.

Tongue tie
This is a birth defect in which the frenulum is short. Babies usually grow out of it before the age of two—speech defects do not occur as a result of this condition. Reassurance is usually all that is required. Occasionally parents may request surgical division.

Macroglossia
Enlargement of the tongue can be seen in acromegaly, Down's syndrome, multiple endocrine adenoma syndrome, hypothyroidism, and amyloidosis.

Burning tongue syndrome
The anterior and lateral aspects of the tongue are most commonly affected and it tends to occur in young women. This is an unsatisfying condition to treat because its cause is unknown and simple analgesics are the only available medications that seem to help.

Hairy leukoplakia
This condition appears as white patches on the lateral border of the tongue, in patients with AIDS.

Black hairy tongue
This aptly named condition occurs due to overgrowth of the filiform papillae of the tongue and generally occurs in smokers. Treatment consists of brushing the tongue with a soft toothbrush.

Ranula
This is a retention cyst which forms in the floor of the mouth under the tongue. It develops from the submandibular or sublingual glands. It is treated by marsupialization.

Cystic hygroma

This is a benign tumour of the lymph vessels (lymphangioma), which consists of large, dilated lymphatic channels. Cystic hygromas usually present at, or soon after, birth, can grow to massive proportions, and may cause life-threatening compression of the airway. They may be injected with sclerosant or surgically exercised.

Tonsillitis

Tonsillitis, or infection of the tonsils, is commonly seen in ENT and in general practice. Common bacterial pathogens are beta-haemolytic streptococci, pneumococci, and *Haemophilus influenzae*. Sometimes tonsillitis occurs following an initial viral infection. Treatment consists of appropriate antibiotics (e.g. penicillin), regular simple analgesia, oral fluids, and bed rest.

Signs of acute tonsillitis
- Sore throat
- Enlargement of the tonsils
- Exudate on the tonsils
- Difficulty in swallowing
- Pyrexia
- Malaise
- Bad breath
- Earache

Complications of tonsillitis

Airway obstruction—is very rare, but may occur in tonsillitis due to glandular fever. The patient may experience severe snoring and acute sleep apnoea, which may require rapid intervention, e.g. insertion of a nasopharyngeal airway or intubation.

Quinsy (peritonsillar abscess)—appears as a swelling of the soft palate and tissues lateral to the tonsil, with displacement of the uvula towards the opposite side. Patients are usually toxic with fetor, trismus, and drooling. Needle aspiration or incision and drainage are required along with antibiotics, which are usually administered intravenously. (☐ See Fig. 23.8, p. 370 and 'How to drain a quinsy', p. 370.)

Parapharyngeal abscess—is a serious complication of tonsillitis and usually presents as a diffuse swelling in the neck. Admission is required and surgical drainage is often necessary via a neck incision. The patient will usually have an ultrasound scan first, to confirm the site and position of the abscess.

Management

Patients with complicated tonsillitis, and those who are unable to drink enough fluid, will need to be admitted to hospital for rehydration, analgesia, and intravenous antibiotics. Ampicillin should be avoided if there is any question of glandular fever, because of the florid skin rash that will occur.

Treatment
(📖 See also 'Tonsillectomy', p. 197.)

Indications for tonsillectomy
Absolute indications for surgery
- Suspected malignancy
- Children with OSA (obstructive sleep apnoea)
- As part of another procedure such as uvulopalatoplasty (UPP) for snoring

Relative indications for surgery
- Recurrent acute tonsillitis
- 3 attacks per year for 3 years, or
- 5 attacks in any one year
- More than one quinsy

Big tonsils which are asymptomatic need not be removed.

Glandular fever

This is also known as 'infectious mononucleosis' or 'Epstein–Barr virus infection'. It is common in teenagers and young adults. Patients with glandular fever may present a similar picture to patients with acute bacterial tonsillitis, but with a slightly longer symptom history. Diagnosis relies upon a positive Monospot or Paul–Bunnell blood test, but early in the course of the disease this test can still show up negative.

Signs and symptoms
- Sore throat
- Pyrexia
- Cervical lymphadenopathy
- White slough on tonsils
- Petechial haemorrhages on the palate
- Marked widespread lymphadenopathy
- Hepatosplenomegaly

Treatment
This is a self-limiting condition for which there is no cure as such. Treatment is largely supportive with painkillers, although patients may appreciate a short course of corticosteroids to decrease swelling. IV fluids may be necessary if they cannot drink enough.

Complications
Patients should be advised to refrain from contact sports for six weeks because of the risk of a ruptured spleen. This can lead to life-threatening internal bleeding.

Tonsillectomy

This is one of the most commonly performed operations. Patients usually stay in hospital for one night, so that bleeding may be recognized and treated appropriately. Tonsils are removed by dissection under general anaesthetic. Haemostasis is achieved with diathermy or ties. (📖 See also Chapter 18, 'Tonsillectomy', p. 318.)

Post-op

Tonsillectomy is very painful and regular simple analgesia is always required afterwards. Patients should be advised that referred pain to the ear is common.

Until the tonsillar fossae are completely healed, eating is very uncomfortable. The traditional jelly and ice cream has now been replaced with crisps, biscuits, and toast, since chewing and swallowing after tonsillectomy is very important for recovery and in helping to prevent infection.

In the immediate postoperative period the tonsillar fossae become coated with a white exudate, which can be mistaken as a sign of infection.

Complications

Postoperative haemorrhage is a serious complication for 5–15% of patients after a tonsillectomy.

A reactive haemorrhage can occur in the first few hours after the operation, this will frequently necessitate a return trip to the operating theatre.

A secondary haemorrhage can occur any time within two weeks of the operation. (📖 See also 'Secondary tonsillar haemorrhage', p. 385.)

Tonsillar tumours

Benign tumours are very rare, but tonsillar stones (tonsiliths) with surrounding ulceration, mucus-retention cysts, herpes simplex, or giant aphthous ulcers, may mimic the more common malignant tumours of the tonsil. These tumours are becoming increasingly common and, unusually, are now being found in younger patients and in non-smokers.

Squamous cell carcinoma (SCC)

This is the commonest tumour of the tonsil. Although it tends to occur in middle-aged and elderly people, in recent years tonsillar SCC has become more frequent in patients under the age of 40. Many of these patients are also unusual candidates for SCC because they are non-smokers and non-drinkers.

Signs and symptoms
• Pain in the throat
• Referred otalgia
• Ulcer on the tonsil
• Lump in the neck

As the tumour grows it may affect the patient's ability to swallow and it may lead to an alteration in the voice—this is known as 'hot potato speech'.

Diagnosis is usually confirmed with a biopsy taken at the time of the staging panendoscopy. FNA of any neck mass is also necessary. Imaging usually entails CT and/or an MRI scan. It is important to exclude any bronchogenic synchronous tumour with a chest X-ray and/or a chest CT scan and bronchoscopy where necessary.

Treatment
Decisions about treatment should be made in a multidisciplinary clinic, taking into account the size and stage of the primary tumour, the presence of nodal metastases, the patient's general medical status, and the patient's wishes.

Treatment options include:
• Radiotherapy alone
• Chemoradiotherapy
• Transoral laser surgery
• En-bloc surgical excision—removes the primary and the affected nodes from the neck. It will often be necessary to reconstruct the surgical defect to allow for adequate speech and swallowing afterwards. This will often take the form of free tissue transfer, such as a radial forearm free flap.

Lymphoma

This is the second most common tonsil tumour.

Signs and symptoms
• Enlargement of one of the tonsils
• Lymphadenopathy in the neck—may be large
• Mucosal ulceration—less common than in SCC

Investigations

- Fine needle aspiration cytology may suggest lymphoma, but it rarely confirms the diagnosis. It is often necessary to perform an excision biopsy of one of the nodes.
- Staging is necessary with CT scanning of the neck chest, abdomen, and pelvis. Further surgical intervention is not required other than to secure a threatened airway.

Treatment

Usually consists of chemotherapy and/or radiotherapy.

Adenoidal enlargement

The adenoid is a collection of loose lymphoid tissue found in the space at the back of the nose. The Eustachian tubes open immediately lateral to the adenoids. Enlargement of the adenoids is very common, especially in children. It may happen as a result of repeated upper respiratory tract infections which occur in children due to their poorly developed immune systems.

Signs and symptoms
- Nasal obstruction
- Nasal quality to the voice
- Mouth breathing which may interfere with eating
- A runny nose
- Snoring
- Obstructive sleep apnoea syndrome (OSAS)
- Blockage of the Eustachian tube

A diagnosis of adenoidal enlargement is usually suspected from the history. Using a mirror or an endoscopic nasal examination will confirm the diagnosis.

The glue ear which arises as a result of poor Eustachian tube function may cause hearing impairment (see 'Glue ear', p. 97). Adenoiditis or infection of the adenoid may allow ascending infections to reach the middle ear via the Eustachian tube.

Treatment
An adenoidectomy is performed under a general anaesthetic. The adenoids are usually removed using suction diathermy or curettage.

Complications
Haemorrhage (primary, reactionary, and secondary)—is a serious complication of adenoidectomy, but is less common than with a tonsillectomy. The procedure is frequently carried out safely as a day case.

Nasal regurgitation—the soft palate acts as a flap valve and separates the nasal and the oral cavity. If the adenoid is removed in patients who have even a minor palatal abnormality, it can have major effects on speech and swallowing. Palatal incompetence can occur in these patients resulting in nasal regurgitation of liquids and nasal escape during speech. Assessment of the palate should form part of the routine ENT examination before such an operation, to avoid this complication.

The salivary glands

Structure and function of the salivary glands

There are three main pairs of salivary glands, the:
- parotid
- submandibular
- sublingual

In addition, a number of other tiny minor salivary glands are scattered throughout the mucosa of the mouth and throat. They produce the saliva needed for digestion and lubricating the food bolus.

The parotid gland

This gland lies on the side of the face or upper neck behind the angle of the mandible and in front of the ear. The gland is pyramid-shaped and covered in thick fibrous tissue. It produces watery, serous saliva. The parotid duct opens into the mouth opposite the second upper molar tooth.

The external carotid artery, retromandibular vein, and lymph nodes all lie within the parotid gland.

The facial nerve traverses the skull base and exits at the stylomastoid foramen. It then passes through the parotid gland splitting into its five main divisions—temporal, zygomatic, buccal, mandibular, cervical—as it does so.

The submandibular gland

This gland lies just below the jaw in front of the angle of the mandible. It produces saliva. The submandibular duct runs from the deep lobe and ends as a papillae, at the front of the floor of the mouth (📖 see Fig. 11.1).

The lingual nerve (which gives sensation to the anterior two-thirds of the tongue) and the hypoglossal nerve (which provides the motor to intrinsic muscles of the tongue) lie in close apposition to the deep surface of the gland.

The marginal mandibular branch of the facial nerve runs just deep to the platysma close under the skin that overlies the gland. Surgeons must be aware of these nerves to prevent iatrogenic damage.

A number of lymph nodes also lie close to or within the submandibular gland.

The sublingual gland

This is the smallest of the major salivary glands. It is found, or felt, in the floor of the mouth, running along the submandibular duct, into which it opens via 10–15 tiny ducts.

Parasympathetic secretor motor supply to the salivary glands

This is rather complicated and is best shown diagrammatically (Fig. 11.2).

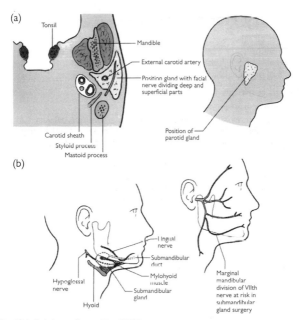

Fig. 11.1 Relations of parotid and SMG.

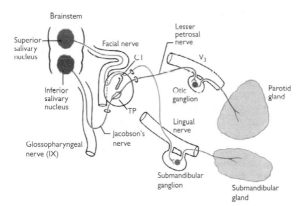

Fig. 11.2 Parasympathetic secretomotor nerve supply.

Salivary gland tumours

- 80% of all salivary gland tumours occur in the parotid gland.
- 80% of these are benign pleomorphic or mixed adenomas.
- 50% of submandibular gland tumours are malignant.
- 80% of minor salivary gland tumours are malignant.

Benign tumours

Pleomorphic adenomas

Parotid pleomorphic adenomas are the most common salivary tumour. They are benign, but if they are present for many years they may turn malignant. They appear most often as an asymptomatic lump behind the angle of the mandible—this may displace the ear lobe upwards slightly. If the patient has weakness of the facial nerve, this suggests a malignant infiltration and the diagnosis must be questioned.

Diagnosis is usually made via FNA, and treatment is surgical. In order to prevent the adenomas recurring, the surgeon should remove a cuff of normal parotid tissue around the lump, and ensure that no tumour is spilt during excision. The surgeon will take great care to identify and preserve the facial nerve during parotid surgery.

Warthin's tumour or adenolymphoma

This is the next most common benign tumour of the salivary glands. It is common in elderly men. It occurs most often in the parotid gland, often in its tail—the part of the parotid that extends into the neck. This is the only tumour which is recognized as occurring bilaterally, and its cause is unknown. Treatment is surgical.

Other benign swellings

These include lipomas, cysts, oncocytomas, and monomorphic adenomas.

Malignant tumours

Malignant salivary gland tumours are much less common than benign ones, but the symptoms can be similar—usually a lump in the neck. The following symptoms may suggest a malignant tumour:

- Pain
- Facial or other nerve weakness
- Skin involvement, such as ulceration or fixation of the overlying skin
- Blood-stained discharge into the mouth
- Local lymph node enlargement suggesting metastasis

Minor salivary glands are present in the mucosa of the nose, mouth, and throat. Neoplastic transformation here is often malignant.

Adenoidcystic tumours (have nothing to do with the adenoids!)

These are the most common malignant salivary gland tumours. They are slow-growing and have a strong tendency to spread along the nerves—this is called 'perineural infiltration'. They can spread several centimetres beyond the palpable lump in this way. Treatment is excision of the tumour and postoperative radiotherapy.

The short-term or 5-year prognosis tends to be good, and patients with a recurrent tumour and even lung metastases may live for years. But the long-term or 25-year prognosis is less good and in most cases patients will eventually die of this disease.

Mucoepidermoid carcinomas

These are unusual tumours in that they have a range of aggressiveness from low to high. High-grade tumours require excision and post-operative radiotherapy, whereas low-grade tumours will usually only need surgery.

Sialadenitis

This is an acute infection of the submandibular or parotid gland. It usually occurs in elderly or debilitated patients, who may be dehydrated and have poor oral hygiene. Drugs, such as the oral contraceptive pill, thiouracil, and alcohol may cause mild sialadenitis.

Signs and symptoms

The symptoms are usually a painful swelling of the gland and pyrexia. Pressure over the affected gland may lead to pus leaking from the duct.

Treatment

Treatment involves rehydration, antibiotics, and attention to oral hygiene. Sialogogues, such as lemon drops which stimulate saliva production, are helpful. Surgical drainage may be required if an intraglandular abscess complicates this infection,

Chronic salivary gland inflammation or recurrent acute attacks of sialadenitis may arise as a result of stones or stricture within the gland or duct. Stones arise as accumulations of calcium and other salts found in saliva, deposits on foreign material, and food debris within the ducts. Strictures most often occur after an episode of inflammation in the duct. Pain and swelling when eating are common. This usually occurs in the submandibular gland, and surgical excision may be required.

Sialolithiasis

Sialolithiasis, or salivary stones, is common, and usually affects the submandibular gland since the secretions are richer in calcium and thicker.

Signs and symptoms

Symptoms may include pain and swelling in the affected gland during or after meals. The gland will become tense and tender. Inspection of the floor of the mouth may reveal the thickened inflamed submandibular duct, and the stone may be palpable within the duct. If there is any uncertainty about the diagnosis, a plain X-ray or a sialogram (an X-ray of the duct system using dye) should be used.

Treatment

Conservative treatment with rehydration, analgesia, and sialogogues may be all that is required. Sometimes a small stone will spontaneously pass out of the duct into the mouth and the symptoms will settle. Larger stones may need to be removed. This can be performed transorally if the stone is palpable in the floor of mouth. If the stone is placed close to the gland, the whole gland may need to be removed by an open operation via the neck.

Other inflammatory conditions

- **Sjögren's syndrome**—is an autoimmune disease. It causes a dry mouth, dry eyes, and in many cases diffuse enlargement of the parotid gland. The diagnosis can be confirmed by biopsying a minor salivary gland found in the mucosa of the oral cavity.
- **Systemic viral infections**—such as mumps and HIV may cause inflammation of the parotid or submandibular glands.
- **Granulomatous conditions**—such as tuberculosis and sarcoidosis may affect the salivary glands.

Pseudosalivary swellings

These swellings may mimic salivary gland enlargement, such as:
- Intraglandular lymph nodes
- Hypertrophy of the masseter muscle—may mimic parotid enlargement
- Parapharyngeal space masses—may present as an intraoral mass in a similar way to a deep lobe of parotid mass
- Lesions/cysts of the mandible or teeth—may look like a submandibular gland mass
- Winging of the mandible—may mimic parotid swelling

Key points—salivary gland swellings

Salivary gland infections and stones	Salivary gland tumours
Usually affect all of the gland	Usually form a lump within part of the gland
Are often painful	Are usually painless unless end-stage malignant
Frequently fluctuate in size	
Become larger and more painful with eating	Usually do not vary in size but grow slowly
Do not lead to cranial nerve palsy	Do not vary with eating
	In association with cranial nerve palsy suggests malignancy

Salivary gland surgery

See figures showing incisions (Fig. 11.3), the facial nerve and its relations to the parotid (Fig. 11.4), and the submandibular gland and anatomy (Fig. 11.5).

The facial nerve passes through the parotid gland—this is a risk in parotid surgery. Surgeons will often use the facial nerve monitor to help them identify the facial nerve.

Other surgical pointers to the position of the facial nerve are listed below:

- The facial nerve **exits** from the stylomastoid foramen which lies at the root of tympanomastoid suture. This is palpable during parotid surgery.
- The facial nerve **lies** approximately 1cm deep and 1cm inferior to a small V-shaped piece of cartilage known as the tragal pointer.
- The facial nerve **bisects** the angle made between the mastoid process and the posterior belly of the digastric muscle.

Complications of parotid gland surgery

- Paraesthesia or numbness of the ear lobe is common, because the greater auricular nerve may need to be divided to gain access to the parotid gland.
- Haematoma.
- Salivary fistula—when saliva leaks out through the incision.
- Temporary facial nerve weakness—occurs in about 10% of cases.
- Permanent facial nerve weakness—occurs in less than 1% of cases.
- Frey's syndrome—sweating and redness of the skin overlying the parotid gland when eating. It occurs when postsynaptic secretomotor nerve fibres are severed during surgery, and they re-grow abnormally, innervating the sweat glands of the skin.

Complications of submandibular gland surgery

- Haematoma—the most common complication.
- Weakness of the marginal mandibular nerve—this can usually be avoided by a low horizontal incision being made 2cm below the angle of the mandible. The surgical dissection should be carried out deep to the capsule of the gland, i.e. in a plane deep to the nerve.
- Lingual and hypoglossal nerve damage—these nerves lie close to the deep surface of the gland and are potentially at risk during the surgery—in reality, damage is extremely rare.

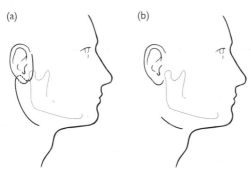

Fig. 11.3 (a) Incision for parotid surgery; (b) incision for submandibular surgery.

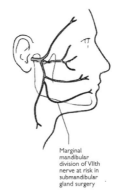

Marginal
mandibular
division of VIIth
nerve at risk in
submandibular
gland surgery

Fig. 11.4 Diagram of facial nerve and relations to the salivary glands.

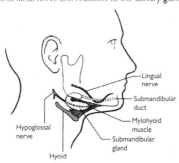

Lingual
nerve

Submandibular
duct

Mylohyoid
muscle

Submandibular
gland

Hypoglossal
nerve

Hyoid

Fig. 11.5 Diagram of submandibular gland and anatomy.

Chapter 12

The larynx

Structure and function of the larynx

Structure

The larynx is a tube made up of cartilage and bone, held together by membranes, ligaments, and muscles. Above, the larynx connects with the pharynx and oral cavity; below, it connects with the trachea and major airways (📖 see Fig. 12.1). Behind the larynx is the opening of the oesophagus.

Food and drink are guided from the mouth to the oesophagus, while air passes via the trachea to the lungs. Food passes over the back of the tongue and runs down two channels called the 'piriform fossae'. These lie slightly behind and to the side of the larynx. They join behind the cricoid cartilage and form the oesophagus (📖 see Fig. 12.2).

Function

The main function of the larynx is to protect the lower airways from contamination by fluids, liquids, and saliva. The way this happens is as follows: the larynx rises during swallowing, bringing the laryngeal inlet closer to the tongue base and allowing the food bolus to pass on either side. The epiglottis folds down to cover the larynx. The vocal cords and false cords (📖 see Fig. 12.3) come together.

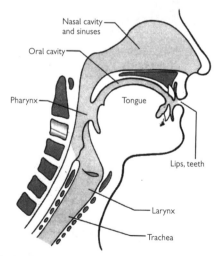

Fig. 12.1 Vocal tract.

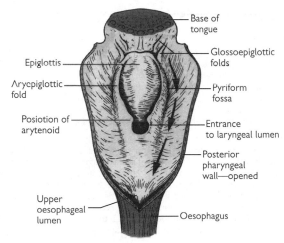

Fig. 12.2 External view of the larynx.

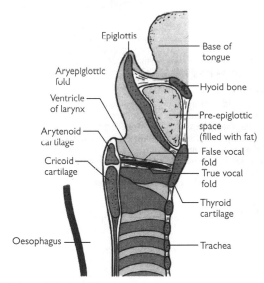

Fig. 12.3 Internal side view of the larynx.

The vocal cords

Structure

The vocal cords, also called the 'vocal folds', and collectively called the 'glottis', are suspended in the airway. They divide the larynx in two—the supraglottis lies above the vocal cords and the subglottis lies below.

The cords are made of a stiff central muscle and ligament, and a soft loose cover. They are fixed to the thyroid cartilage at the front and to the arytenoid cartilages at the back. These cartilages can slide away from and towards each other, opening and closing the laryngeal inlet.

Innervation

The sensation of the supraglottis is carried by the internal branch of the superior laryngeal nerve. The external branch carries motor fibres to the cricothyroid muscle. This muscle is important in adjusting the tension of the vocal cord. The vagus nerve gives rise to the recurrent laryngeal nerve, and this in turn carries sensation to the subglottis and is motor to all the other muscles of the larynx. The left recurrent laryngeal nerve has an unusually long course and loops down into the chest, lying close to the hilum of the lung. It is prone to infiltration by tumours of this region. (☐ See Fig. 12.8.)

Lymph drainage

The vocal cords are a watershed for lymphatic drainage. Above, the supraglottis drains to the pre-epiglottic and upper deep cervical nodes; below, drainage is to the lower deep cervical and pretracheal nodes. The cords have very poor lymph drainage, so tumours limited to vocal cords have a low risk of lymphatic spread. Tumours of the lymphatic-rich supra- or subglottis frequently present with lymph node metastases and consequently will have a worse prognosis (Fig. 12.4).

Function

The vocal cords are the source of the sound vibration, which we adapt with our mouth, tongue, lips, and teeth to produce speech. As air passes up between the cords the Bernoulli effect draws the mucosa of the cords together. They meet for a fraction of a second and then the pressure rises below the cords, blowing them apart again. This vibration of the cords and the distortion of the mucosa that results from it is known as the 'mucosal wave'. This causes the voice.

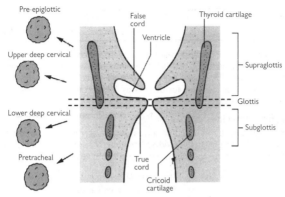

Fig. 12.4 Lymph drainage of the larynx.

Congenital laryngeal lesions

Babies are more prone to breathing difficulties because their larynx differs from an adult's in the following ways:

- The airway is smaller both relatively and absolutely.
- The laryngeal mucosa is less tightly bound down and as a result may swell dramatically.
- The cartilaginous support for the airway is less rigid than in an adult—this makes it more prone to collapse, especially during inspiration.

Laryngomalacia

Signs of this condition show themselves shortly after birth with inspiratory stridor and feeding difficulties. When breathing in, these babies experience an excessive collapse and indrawing of the supraglottic airways, leading to breathing difficulties.

Usually this condition is mild and self-limiting. When it is severe an aryepiglottoplasty may be performed. This involves dividing the excessively tight aryepiglottic folds, which allows the epiglottis to spring upwards and open up the airway.

Subglottic stenosis

This abnormality is caused by an excessively narrow cricoid cartilage. It is either a birth defect, or it arises as a result of intubation and prolonged ventilation. Subglottic cysts and haemangiomas may present with similar symptoms.

The main sign of this condition is stridor at any age from birth to 2 years. Diagnosis is made by inspecting and measuring the diameter of the subglottis under general anaesthetic. Mild cases may be treated conservatively, but more severe stenoses require surgical invervention and laryngotracheal reconstruction. 📖 See Table 12.1 for Cotton grading of stenosis.

Laryngeal web

This condition occurs when the vocal cords fuse together and the airway is reduced. Fusion can be minimal, with little effect on the airway; or complete fusion can occur which is incompatible with life.

The main signs of this condition are respiratory difficulties, stridor, and a hoarse cry. Severe cases will require immediate surgical intervention, either via a tracheostomy (when an artificial breathing hole is made in the neck below the cords to bypass the obstruction) or by endoscopic division of the web.

Laryngeal cleft

This condition occurs when the posterior larynx has failed to fuse. At its most severe this will also extend down to involve the posterior wall of the trachea.

The main signs are respiratory problems associated with feeding, as a result of aspiration into the trachea. However, mild cases can be difficult to diagnose. Where there are symptoms, surgical repair may be needed.

Vocal cord palsy

The recurrent laryngeal nerves are long in children and adults, reaching from the skull base down into the chest and back up again to the larynx. Because of their length, they are prone to damage anywhere along their course. Unilateral palsy will cause a weak breathy cry and feeding difficulties as a result of aspiration, and bilateral palsy will present as marked stridor.

Table 12.1 Congenital laryngeal lesions: cotton grading of tracheal stenosis

Grade 1	≤50% obstruction
Grade 2	51–70% obstruction
Grade 3	71–99% obstruction
Grade 4	No lumen

Infections of the larynx

Acute laryngitis

Inflammation of the larynx may occur in isolation or as part of a general infective process affecting the whole of the respiratory tract. It is very common, often presenting as a sore throat and loss of voice with a cold.

Signs and symptoms
- Hoarse voice
- Pain on speaking and swallowing
- Malaise
- Slight pyrexia
- Examination of the vocal cords will show them to be reddened and swollen

Treatment

Most patients with acute laryngitis either self-medicate or are treated in the primary care setting with supportive therapy such as voice rest, simple analgesia, steam inhalations, and simple cough suppressants.

Voice rest is especially important for any professional voice user. Patients should be advised of this, and of the risk of haemorrhage into the vocal cord, which can produce permanent adverse effects on the voice.

Chronic laryngitis

Chronic laryngitis is a common inflammation of the larynx caused by many different factors. It often begins after an upper respiratory tract infection. Smoking, vocal abuse, chronic lung disease, sinusitis, postnasal drip, reflux, alcohol fumes, and environmental pollutants may all conspire together to maintain the inflammation.

Signs and symptoms
- A hoarse voice.
- A tickle in the throat or a feeling of mucus in the throat.
- A patient who is constantly clearing their throat or coughing—this causes still more inflammation of the cords and establishes a vicious circle.
- A laryngoscopy which reveals thickened, red, oedematous vocal cords.

The patient should be referred for a laryngeal examination if their symptoms fail to settle within 4 weeks. If any concern remains after this examination, the patient should be admitted for an examination and a biopsy, under general anaesthetic, to exclude laryngeal malignancy.

Treatment

Any agents that are causing the chronic laryngitis should be removed. The patient may require the skills of a speech therapist. Patients will also respond well to explanation and reassurance that they do not have a more serious condition.

Reinke's oedema

This is a specific form of chronic laryngitis found in smokers. The vocal cords become extremely oedematous and filled with a thin jelly-like fluid. The oedema fails to resolve due to poor lymph drainage of the vocal cord. Stopping smoking and speech therapy are helpful in removing the causes of this condition. In many cases microlaryngeal surgery is required to incise the cord and suck out the oedema. It is important to avoid any damage to the free edge of the vocal cord when performing this operation, as it can permanently affect the mucosal wave and hence the voice.

Epiglottitis and supraglottitis

This is an inflammation of the epiglottis or supraglottic tissues that affects children and adults. Epiglottitis is now rare in children in the UK (as a result of the haemophilus influenza type b (HIB) vaccination). It is seen more often in adults, where it tends to affect the whole of the supraglottic tissues (and is called 'supraglottitis'). Most ENT departments see one case per month in the winter.

The causative agent is usually *Haemophilus influenzae*.

Signs and symptoms
- Difficulty in swallowing leading to drooling of saliva.
- Change in the voice, described as a muffled or 'hot potato voice' or change in the child's cry.
- Dramatic swelling of the supraglottic tissues.
- Pools of saliva seen collected around the larynx on endoscopy.

This condition should not be underestimated. It may start with features similar to any other respiratory tract infection, but it can rapidly progress to total airway obstruction within hours of onset. Consider this diagnosis early on, and get expert help.

Management
- Admit the patient and keep them upright. Laying the patient flat could obstruct their airway.
- Do not attempt to examine the mouth, as this may obstruct the patient's breathing.
- No X-rays—they do not add much to the diagnosis and remove the patient from immediate expert assistance should they need it.
- Call for senior help—an ENT surgeon and an anaesthetist.

Treatment

If epiglottitis or supraglottitis is suspected, stop further investigations. Escort the patient calmly and quickly to an operating theatre where an experienced paediatric anaesthetist and scrubbed consultant ENT surgeon are standing by with the appropriate equipment (laryngoscope, ventilating bronchoscope, and tracheostomy set).

Where possible, the patient should be intubated and treated with the appropriate antibiotics. However, oral intubation may be difficult and the ENT surgeon may be asked to secure the airway surgically.

Croup

This infection is common in children. It affects the whole of the upper respiratory tract (URT), hence the more descriptive name, 'acute laryngotracheobronchitis'. It is usually viral in origin, but a bacterial infection with *H. influenzae* is sometimes seen. The speed of onset of croup is slower than in epiglottitis, but it can be extremely serious and even life-threatening.

Signs and symptoms
- Mild preceding upper respiratory tract infection
- Rising pyrexia
- Stridor
- Malaise

Treatment
- Admission to hospital may be necessary in all but the most minor cases
- Intravenous antibiotics
- Nebulized adrenaline
- Ventilatory support where required

Cancer of the larynx

The vast majority of laryngeal cancers are squamous cell carcinomas. Smoking is the risk factor for laryngeal cancer, although smoking and drinking in combination puts the patient at even more risk. It is the most common neck and head malignancy.

Since the whole of the upper aerodigestive tract has been exposed to the same risk factor (that is, smoke), there is a widespread field change throughout this mucosa. These patients therefore have an increased risk of developing another cancer in the mouth, pharynx, larynx, or oesophagus. Some 5% of patients with one head and neck cancer will present with a second primary tumour elsewhere in the head or neck. This may be silent and cause no symptoms at all!

Signs and symptoms

The patient's symptoms will depend upon which site(s) within the larynx is affected. A tumour on the vocal cord will cause a hoarse voice, and a patient in this situation will usually present early. However, a tumour in the supraglottis may present few symptoms until much later and a patient may present with advanced disease. All patients with a lump in the neck must be referred for an ENT examination.

Signs of advanced laryngeal cancer are:
- Pain—often referred to the ear
- Voice change—the voice is muffled rather than hoarse, unless the tumour also extends to involve the true vocal cords
- Breathing difficulties and stridor
- Difficulty swallowing or inhaling
- Lymph node enlargement in the neck—this is often the only presenting feature

Investigations

Although a clinical diagnosis can often be made after examination of the larynx, a biopsy is essential. This is because conditions such as laryngeal papillomas, granulomas, and polyps may mimic laryngeal cancer. All patients should also undergo examination of the whole of the upper aerodigestive tract (panendoscopy) to check for a second primary tumour.

All patients must have at least a CXR. A CT scan of the chest is routine practice in many centres. CT/MRI scanning of the neck is also mandatory, particularly looking for thyroid cartilage erosion and enlarged lymph nodes in the deep cervical chain.

Staging

TNM staging is applied to head and neck cancers in a similar way to other sites (☐ see Boxes 12.1–12.3):
- The T stage is determined by the anatomical site/sites affected.
- The N stage refers to the local nodal spread.
- The M stage is determined by the presence or absence of distant metastases.

Box 12.1 T staging of laryngeal cancer

TX: Tumour cannot be assessed.

Tis: Carcinoma *in situ*.

T1a: Tumour limited to one cord and not affecting the anterior commisure.

T1b: Tumour limited to the cord but involving the anterior (or posterior) commisure.

T2:   Tumour spreading upwards or downwards from the cord to involve the supraglottis or subglottis with normal vocal cord mobility.

T3:   Tumour which fixes the vocal cord either by involvement of the recurrent laryngeal nerve or by infiltration of the cricoarytenoid joint, or simply as a result of the bulk of the tumour.

T4:   Tumour escaping from the larynx to involve another site or erosion of the cartilaginous framework of the larynx.

Box 12.2 N staging for the head and neck

N1:   A single ipsilateral node <3cm in size.

N2a: A single ipsilateral node >3cm but <6cm in size.

N2b: More than one ipsilateral node <6cm in size.

N2c: A contralateral node or bilateral nodes <6cm in size.

N3:   Any node >6cm in size.

Box 12.3 M staging for the head and neck

M0:   No distant metastases.

M1:   Distant metastases.

Treatment of laryngeal cancer

Treatment is with surgery or external beam radiotherapy. Early laryngeal tumours are satisfying to treat, since more than 90% can be cured.

If a patient is too unfit to undergo radical treatment, palliative radiotherapy or chemotherapy may be used to shrink the tumour. This can reduce symptoms and improve the patient's quality of life.

Although practice does vary slightly between different units and countries, in general, treatment is as follows:

- Small tumours (stage T1 and T2) are treated with radiotherapy—surgery is used only if they recur afterwards.
- Big tumours (stage T4) are treated with radical excision—a partial or total laryngectomy.
- The treatment of T3 tumours is controversial—some opt for primary surgery and others advocate radiotherapy, holding surgery in reserve for radiation failures.

Each patient should be assessed individually and treatment decisions must be made in a multidisciplinary team setting, with the knowledge and consent of the patient.

Surgery for laryngeal cancer

The decision as to which type of surgery is performed largely depends on the size and extent of the tumour. Surgery may either be performed endoluminally—with endoscopes from the inside—usually with the aid of a laser, or the radical excision of part of, or the entire, larynx may be needed. In general, smaller tumours (T1 and T2) are more easily treated with endoscopic laser surgery, and patients with larger T3 and 4 tumours are offered radical excisional surgery. (📖 See 'Laryngectomy', p. 227.)

Radical radiotherapy for laryngeal cancer (Box 12.4)

A total dose of 50–70Gy is given over 4–6 weeks, Monday to Friday.

Each treatment only lasts a few minutes but the patient has to wear a custom-made Perspex mask, rather like a neck brace. This holds the patient in exactly the same position each day, ensuring that the radiotherapy fields are directed accurately onto the tumour and immediate area. This spares the uninvolved areas of the head and neck.

Towards the end of treatment the patient will suffer with painful mucositis. Swallowing can become difficult, and the patient may need to be admitted for enteral feeding and analgesia.

Box 12.4 Key points—radiotherapy for laryngeal cancer

- Treatment intent may be palliative or curative.
- Chemotherapy is only used as an addition to radiotherapy (or surgical) treatment.
- Small tumours do very well.
- Radiotherapy is usually given for small tumours.
- Large tumours are usually treated with a laryngectomy.
- Postoperative radiotherapy is often given in advanced disease with poor histology.

Laryngectomy

Several different types of partial laryngectomy have been described. These are collectively known as 'less than total' and are beyond the scope of this book.

Total laryngectomy

This was first described at the beginning of the last century, but it remains a reliable and effective treatment. During a total laryngectomy the larynx is removed and the trachea is brought to the skin as an end-stoma in the neck. The pharynx is opened and repaired to reconstitute the swallowing mechanism (Fig. 12.5). A neck dissection is often performed in combination with this procedure. This is because patients with advanced or recurrent laryngeal disease are at considerable risk of having nodal metastases, which may either be palpable or hidden.

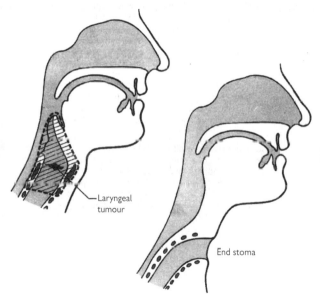

Laryngeal tumour

End stoma

Fig. 12.5 Diagram of pre- and postlaryngectomy anatomy.

Voice restoration after laryngectomy (📖 see also 'Speech and language therapists', p. 343.)

Oesophageal speech (📖 see Fig. 12.6a)

In those who can achieve it, oesophageal speech offers near-normal verbal communication. The basic principle is that air is swallowed into the stomach and then regurgitated into the pharynx. This causes vibration of the pharyngo-oesophageal segment (PE segment) similar to a belch. This can be modified with the lips and teeth into intelligible speech.

The main problem is that not all patients can manage to achieve this type of speech, and even if they do, only small amounts of air can be swallowed. This means that the resultant speech can only be made up of short phrases at best.

Tracheo-oesophageal puncture (📖 see Fig. 12.6b)

This is when artificial communication is created between the back wall of the trachea and the front wall of the pharynx/oesophagus. This is usually done at the time of the initial surgery (primary puncture) but can be performed at anytime thereafter (secondary puncture).

A one-way valve is inserted into this tract which allows the passage of air from the trachea to the oesophagus, vibrating the PE segment as above. In order to activate the valve, the patient must occlude their stoma and try to breathe out. This may be done with a finger, or by using a second manually operated valve which sits over the stoma as part of a heat and moisture exchanger (HME). The HME also filters the inhaled air and prevents excess water vapour being lost from the respiratory tract—in effect this replaces some of the functions of the nose.

Artificial larynx (Servox)

Some patients cannot achieve either of the above forms of speech, and require an external vibrating source. The vibrating end of this device is held firmly onto the patient's neck, floor of their mouth or cheek, and this causes these tissues to vibrate. As a result, the air within the pharynx and oral cavity vibrates and sound is produced. The voice produced does sound rather unnatural but this is a simple and effective means of communication (📖 see Fig. 12.7).

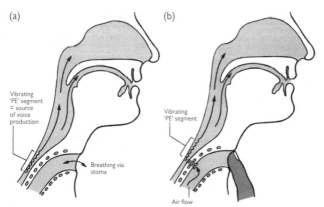

Fig. 12.6 Diagram of TEP voice.

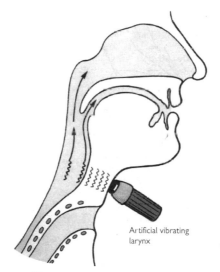

Fig. 12.7 Diagram of Servox.

Benign lesions of the larynx

These are lesions of the vocal cords which are not cancer. Signs of a benign lesion—such as a hoarse voice—can be indistinguishable from those of laryngeal cancer. It is therefore imperative that any patient with a change in their voice lasting more that 4 weeks is referred to an ENT surgeon to exclude a laryngeal malignancy.

Vocal cord polyp/cyst

These lesions are indistinguishable histologically from each other. They usually arise spontaneously, but may be associated with previous laryngeal inflammation. Symptoms are a sore throat and/or a hoarse voice.

The cysts are intracordal, whereas polyps are pedunculated and may be difficult to see because they sometimes hang down on their stalk to sit below the cords. Treatment is with microsurgical excision, taking care to avoid iatrogenic damage to the free edge of the vocal cord, and hence the mucosal wave and voice.

Vocal cord granuloma

This lesion is usually unilateral and affects the posterior aspect of the vocal cord. As a result, it can have quite a minimal effect on the voice. Vocal cord granuloma arises as a result of inflammation of the arytenoid cartilage (perichondritis). It is most often seen as a result of intubation trauma or excessive coughing. The patient usually complains of pain in their larynx. Reflux is a commonly associated feature.

The lesion requires a biopsy as SCC can present with similar features. Treatment may include surgical excision, speech therapy, and the treatment of acid reflux.

Singer's nodules

These nodules—also known as 'screamers' nodules'—occur as a result of prolonged voice abuse or misuse. They are common in children, amateur actors, and singers—they give a characteristic huskiness to the voice.

They are always bilateral and occur at the junction of the anterior one-third and posterior two-thirds of the vocal cords. Early or 'soft' nodules will resolve with speech therapy and good vocal habits, but long-established 'hard' nodules may require surgery.

Papillomata

These non-cancerous growths are most commonly seen in children, but may also occur in adults. Papillomas arise as a result of HPV (human papillomavirus) infection. The route of transmission is thought to be through inhalation. There may also be some defect in the host immune system, as some individuals are affected and others are not. Spontaneous resolution tends to occur in children around puberty, but this is less common in adults.

In its most severe form, a papilloma may result in significant airway obstruction in the larynx, trachea, and major bronchii. If the patient's airway is obstructed, surgical debulking of the papilloma is required. Removal of every last papilloma is not advised, since this will cause scarring of the vocal cords and they often recur. A tracheostomy may be required, but even then papillomas may grow around the stoma.

Malignant transformation may occur in adults, especially with subtypes 7 and 11. Systemic treatment with interferon is effective, but rebound growth may be dramatic when it is stopped.

Muscle tension dysphonia

This is a common problem seen in general and ENT practice. Symptom is a hoarse voice which tires easily and may vary in pitch. Patients sometimes say their voice 'cracks' or 'gives out' and the quality of the voice varies from day to day and moment to moment. Occasionally the patient may present with aphonia.

These problems are caused by laryngeal muscular tension abnormalities. They are associated with voice misuse, psychological stress, and psychiatric disease.

Globus-type symptoms are frequent. These include a feeling of a lump in the throat, a feeling of mucus in the throat, and frequent throat clearing. The treatment is reassurance and explanation, with speech therapy for patients who do not respond well.

Vocal cord palsy

Palsy or paralysis of the vocal cords will mean that the patient may have a weak breathy voice rather than the harsh hoarse voice of laryngeal cancer. They will have a poor, ineffective cough and aspiration is common. (📖 See Box 12.5.)

The recurrent laryngeal nerve (RLN) is a branch of the vagus nerve and has a long course (📖 see Fig. 12.8). This makes it susceptible to damage in a variety of sites.

Investigation

Remember the rule of thirds below:
- $1/3$ idiopathic
- $1/3$ surgery
- $1/3$ neoplasia

Where there is no history of recent surgery, order:
- CXR—if it is negative proceed to:
- CT scan—skull base to hilum
- ± USS thyroid
- ± oesphagoscopy

If the above are negative then postviral neuropathy is the most likely cause. The causes of vocal cord immobility (fixation rather than palsy) include rheumatoid arthritis, laryngeal trauma, prolonged intubation, and carcinoma affecting the cricoarytenoid joint. An endoscopy, together with palpation of the joint, is necessary to confirm this abnormality.

Treatment

Where there is a small gap between the cords, speech therapy may be all that is needed to strengthen the mobile cord and aid compensation. When there is a larger gap, the paralysed cord can be medialized, either by an injection technique or via a thyroplasty (📖 see Figs 12.10 and 12.11). Poor function of the cords may lead to aspiration and chest infections. Dietary modifications, tube feeding, and even a tracheostomy may be required to protect the airway from soiling.

Neurological laryngeal conditions

Any condition which affects the brainstem (CVA, trauma, or tumour) will affect the function of the vagus nerve, and as such the recurrent laryngeal nerve. With these conditions, the voice problems may be less a cause for concern than the lack of protection of the airway, which can lead to life-threatening aspiration. Any systemic neurological or neuromuscular condition, such as multiple sclerosis or muscular dystrophy, may also affect the voice. But it is rare for these conditions to present first to an ENT surgeon as voice problems.

Box 12.5 Learning points—vocal cord palsy

- Unilateral vocal cord palsy leads to vocal cord lateralization and a weak voice but a good airway.
- Bilateral vocal cord palsy leads to vocal cord medialization and airway problems but a good voice.

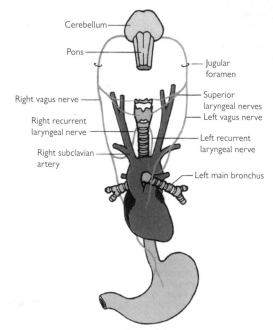

Fig. 12.8 Diagram of RLN anatomy and sites of damage.

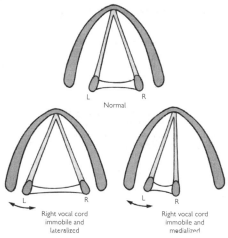

Fig. 12.9 Diagram of palsy positions.

L   R
Normal

L   R
Right vocal cord
immobile and
lateralized

L   R
Right vocal cord
immobile and
medialized

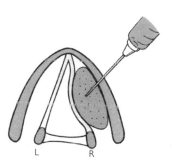

Fig. 12.10 Diagram of injection.

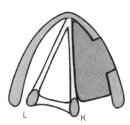

Fig. 12.11 Diagram of thyroplasty.

Differential diagnosis of a hoarse voice

Voice problems are common: the majority are due to URTI and will settle with little or simple supportive treatment. However, failure to improve should raise the suspicion of laryngeal pathology and any patient with constant hoarse voice (i.e. where the voice never returns to normal) for more than 4 week should be referred urgently to the ENT clinic for laryngoscopy in order to examine the vocal cords and exclude a laryngeal cancer or other pathology. Many patients will present with a minor and fluctuating hoarseness and here the most likely diagnosis is a muscle tension or functional dysphonia. The problem is usually well treated with a course of speech therapy. The important and common causes of vocal problems and the most typical features are shown in Table 12.2 p. 235.

Table 12.2 Common causes of dysphonia

Diagnosis	Voice quality	Duration	Special features	Treatment
Laryngeal cancer	Hoarse/gruff	Constant >4/52 progressive	Smoking history Neck lump? Referred otalgia	RT/surgery
Vocal cord palsy	Weak/breathy Poor 'bovine' cough	Constant >4/52	Smoking history. Frequently due to lung cancer	Exclude lung cancer. Consider thyroplasty to improve the voice
Vocal cord nodules	Husky	Usually variable	Poor singing technique, shouting, or voice abuse	Speech and language therapist (SALT), rarely surgery
Functional dysphonia	Mildly husky	Varies, i.e. periods when the voice is normal	Voice tires easily, worse in the evenings, often associated with stress/life events	SALT & reassurance
Reinke's oedema	Gruff and deep. Women often say they sound like a man	Constant—non-progressive	Smoking history hypothyroid	Stop smoking SALT Surgery
Neurological causes	Variable, difficulty with pitch control. Often associated also with dysarthria	Variable	Other neurological signs & symptoms. Frequently also mild dysphagia	Refer to neurology SALT

Stridor

Stridor is a high-pitched noise caused by a restricted airway. It is most common in children, due to the anatomical differences between the paediatric and the adult larynx (□ see 'Congenital laryngeal lesions', p. 218).

The timing of the stridor in respiration tells you the obstruction or restriction site:

- Laryngeal stridor = inspiratory
- Tracheal stridor = expiratory—a wheeze
- Subglottic stridor = biphasic—occurs when breathing in or out

A small reduction in the diameter of the airway leads to a dramatic increase in the airway resistance and hence the work of breathing (Poiseuille's law of resistance = r^4).

Causes of stridor

Congenital

- Laryngomalacia
- Vocal cord web
- Bilateral vocal cord palsy
- Subglottic stenosis

Acquired

- Trauma
- Foreign body
- Epiglottitis/supraglottitis
- Croup
- Carcinoma
- Airway compression, e.g. thyroid

Assessment

Stridor is an ominous sign. Even if the patient appears to be coping, be sure that they are closely observed and that facilities to secure the airway are readily at hand. Patients may suddenly decompensate with devastating consequences.

- Take a rapid history
- Measure O_2 saturation
- Take temperature
- Check respiratory rate

In children, pyrexia, drooling, dysphagia, and a rapid progression of the illness, suggests epiglottitis. Take the patient to a place of safety such as a resuscitation room or operating theatre, and call for a senior ENT surgeon and experienced anaesthetist.

A similar history in adults suggests supraglottitis. This diagnosis can usually be confirmed by a careful nasolaryngoscopy. (□ See also 'The emergency airway', p. 237.)

The emergency airway

Remember to keep calm!
  The following questions should be answered first:
- Will admission and observation be sufficient for the time being, or do you need to intervene to secure the airway?
- If intervention is required do you need to do something now, or do you have time to wait for senior help to arrive?

Assessment

Assessment should follow three stages—Look, listen, and observe.

Look
- What is the patient's colour—are they blue?
- Is there any intercostal recession or tracheal tug?
- What is the patient's respiratory rate?

Listen
- Can the patient talk in sentences, phrases, words, or not at all?
- Do they have stridor? Is it inspiratory, expiratory, or mixed?
- What history can the patient give?

Observation
- Is the patient's respiratory rate climbing?
- Is the patient feverish?
- What is the patient's O_2 saturation? Is it falling?

Interventions

Consider the following options:
- Oxygen via a face mask or nasal prongs
- Broad-spectrum antibiotics, such as co-amoxiclav (check the patient is not allergic)
- Nebulized adrenaline (1ml of 1:1000 with 1ml saline)
- Heliox—this is a mixture of helium and oxygen that is less dense than air. It is easier to breathe, and it buys you time, during which you can take steps to stabilize the airway

Endotracheal intubation

This should be the first line of intervention where possible. If it proves difficult or impossible, move on quickly.

Tracheostomy

A surgical hole is made in the trachea below the cords. In an emergency, a longitudinal incision is made in the midline of the neck and deepened to the trachea, dividing the thyroid. Brisk bleeding is to be expected. The blade is plunged into the airway and twisted sideways to hold the tracheal fenestration open. A cuffed tracheostomy or ET tube is inserted into the airway and the bleeding thyroid is dealt with afterwards.

Cricothyroidotomy

☐ See Fig. 12.13.

Indications

Upper airway obstruction when endotracheal intubation is not possible, e.g. irretrievable foreign body, facial oedema (burns, angio-oedema), maxillofacial trauma, infection (epiglottitis).

Procedure

- Lie the patient supine with their neck extended.
- Run your index finger down the neck anteriorly in the midline. First you will find the notch in the upper border of the thyroid cartilage (the Adam's apple). Just below this you will come to a depression—the cricothyroid membrane which feels slightly spongy. It lies just above the prominence of the cricoid cartilage.

NB: Needle and Mini-Trach® are temporary measures pending formal tracheostomy.

1 *Emergency needle cricothyroidotomy:*

- Pierce the membrane with a large-bore cannula (14G) attached to a syringe: withdrawal of air confirms position; lidocaine may or may not be required.
- Advance the cannula at 45° to the skin superiorly in the sagittal plane.
- Use a Y-connector or improvised connection to the O_2 supply at 15L/min: use your thumb on the Y-connector to allow O_2 in over 1s and CO_2 out over 4s ('transtracheal jet insufflation'). This is the preferred method in children <12yrs. However, this will only sustain life for 30–45min before CO_2 builds up.

2 *Mini-Trach II®:*

- This contains a guarded blade, introducer, 4mm uncuffed tube (slide over introducer) with ISO connection and binding tape.
- The patient will have to be ventilated via a bag, as the resistance is too high to breathe spontaneously.
- This will sustain life for 30–45min.

3 *Surgical cricothyroidotomy:*

- Smallest tube for prolonged ventilation is 6mm.
- Introduce high-volume, low-pressure cuff tracheostomy tube through a horizontal incision in the membrane. Take care not to cut the cricoid cartilage.

Complications

- Local haemorrhage
- Aspiration
- Posterior perforation of the trachea ± oesophagus
- Subglottic stenosis if the cricoid is damaged
- Tube blockage
- Tube misplacement due to anterior subcutaneous tunnelling

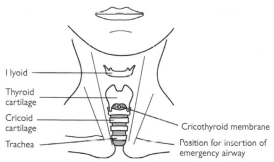

Fig. 12.12 Cricothyroidotomy.

Further reading

This section is substantially based on the advice to be found in the *Oxford Handbook of Clinical Medicine*, 7th edition, Oxford University Press, and is used with thanks.

Tracheostomy care and trache tubes

Tracheostomy operation

In an elective tracheostomy, the incision is usually placed horizontally. The strap muscles are separated in the midline, and the thyroid isthmus is carefully divided and oversewn. The trachea is opened at the 3rd or 4th tracheal ring, and a window of tracheal cartilage is removed. A tracheostomy tube of the right size (three-quarters of the diameter of the trachea) is inserted and the cuff is inflated.

Tracheostomy tubes (□ See Figs 12.13 and 12.14.)

The choice of tubes may seem bewildering, but the basic principles are as follows:

Trache tubes with inner tubes

The inner tube is slightly longer than the outer, and crusting tends to occur at the distal end and on the inner tube. The inner tube can easily be removed, cleaned, and replaced without removing the outer tube. Any patient who is likely to require a tracheostomy for more than 1 week is probably best fitted with a trache tube with an inner.

Cuffed and non-cuffed tubes

The cuff, as in an endotracheal tube, is high volume and low pressure. This prevents damage to the tracheal wall. The cuff prevents fluid and saliva leaking around the tube and into the lungs. In addition, it makes an airtight seal between the tube and the trachea, so allowing for positive pressure ventilation. Most tubes are cuffed, but when a tracheostomy is in place long term, a non-cuffed tube may be used to prevent damage to the trachea.

Metal tubes

Metal tubes are non-cuffed and are used only for patients with permanent tracheostomies. They have the advantage of being inert and 'speaking valves' can be inserted.

Fenestrated tubes

Most tubes are non-fenestrated. The advantage of a fenestrated tube (one with a hole in its side wall) is that air can pass through the fenestration, through the vocal cords, and enable the patient to talk. The disadvantage is that saliva and liquids may penetrate through the fenestration into the lower respiratory tree.

Post-tracheostomy care

In the first few days after a tracheostomy operation, special care needs to be taken. The patient should be nursed by staff familiar with tracheostomy care. The patient should be given a pad and pencil with which to communicate.

Precautions

- The tube should be secured with tapes, and knotted at the side of the neck until a tract is well established.
- The tapes should be tied with the neck slightly flexed.

- Cuff should not be over-inflated—to prevent ischaemic damage to the tracheal wall. Use a pressure gauge to check the cuff's pressure.
- The patient must be given humidification for at least the first 48h to reduce tracheal crusting.
- Regular suctioning of the airway to clear secretions may be needed.
- A spare tracheostomy tube and an introducer should be kept by the patient's bed in case of accidental displacement of the tube.
- Tracheal dilators should also be close by for the same reason.

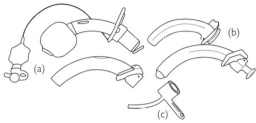

Fig. 12.13 Diagram of tracheostomy tubes (a) Cuffed fenestrated tube; (b) non–cuffed, non-fenestrated tube; (c) paediatric tube.

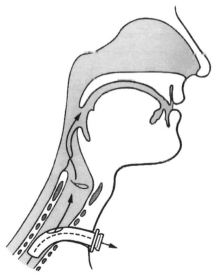

Fig. 12.14 Diagram of tracheostomy tube position (note fenestration).

The oesophagus

Introduction

The oesophagus is a muscular tube connecting the pharynx to the stomach. In adults it is 25cm long. It starts at the level of C6, the cricoid cartilage, and it ends at the gastro-oesophageal junction, or the diaphragm. The cricopharyngeus muscle acts as an upper oesophageal sphincter.

Congenital oesophageal conditions

These rare conditions may account for some cases of ↑ infant death, feeding problems, or failure to thrive. They are frequently associated with other abnormalities of the larynx and/or the trachea. Complex surgery may be required and treatment should be given in specialist paediatric centres (🕮 see Fig. 13.1).

Oesophageal foreign bodies

(🕮 See p. 384.)

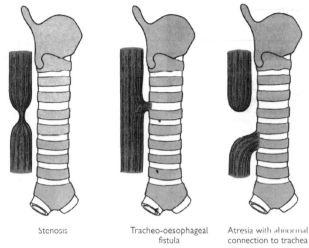

Stenosis   Tracheo-oesophageal   Atresia with abnormal
                fistula   connection to trachea

Fig. 13.1 Congenital oesophageal lesions.

Globus

Globus pharyngeus/syndrome/hystericus are all terms which have been used to describe a common symptom complex of a 'feeling of a lump in the throat (FOSIT) with no obvious cause'. It is probably caused by excess muscle tension in the pharyngeal musculature.

Features include
- Feeling of a lump in the throat
- Mucus collection in the throat which is rarely cleared
- Symptoms come and go
- Symptoms are usually in the midline
- The sensation is most noted when swallowing saliva rather than food or drink
- Worse when stressed
- Worse when tired
- More common in women
- Associated with GORD

Pharyngeal malignancy may present with similar symptoms, so beware especially:
- Unilateral globus
- Globus and otalgia
- Globus and a neck lump
- Persistent/progressive symptoms

Reassurance is usually all that is required to treat globus, but barium swallow or endoscopy may be required to exclude malignant disease.

Chronic cough/throat clearing/laryngeal spasm

Patients present with a myriad of throat symptoms, many of which do not conform to the major pathological processes outlined in this and other textbooks. The most common of these symptoms are:

- Irritation
- Tickle
- Cough
- Throat clearing
- A sensation of mucus in the throat
- Choking

In the vast majority of cases there is little to find on ENT examination, nevertheless it is mandatory in order to exclude more serious disease. Most patients can be easily managed via reassurance and careful explanation that the throat is a very sensitive area and the cough reflex is a natural protective reflex which can become 'upregulated' when a source of irritation is present. It is important to explore the sorts of likely laryngopharyngeal irritants in their particular case, identification of which will require direct questioning within the history.

Common causes of laryngopharyngeal irritation

Reflux
Acidic stomach contents may pass upwards to the throat. Not surprisingly, this causes an irritation in the throat as a result of a low-level chemical burn.

Mouth breathing and blocked nose
The nose is the air-conditioning unit for the lower airways. It warms and moistens the air we breathe very effectively. If the nose is blocked and mouth breathing takes over then this effect is lost and the throat and airways soon become dry and sensitive.

Rhinitis
Rhinitis can lead to throat problems, either due to a partial blocking of the nose (see above), or due to postnasal drip. This is the production of excessive nasal mucus which can drip into the throat causing irritation and excessive swallowing.

Asthma and lung disease
Many patients with rhinitis also have asthma, and vice versa. It is not surprising that people with a sensitivity of the upper airway (rhinitis) and/or of the lower airway (asthma) often have a sensitivity of the area in between, i.e. the throat. Other lung conditions, such as bronchitis, can lead to an excessive production of mucus in the lungs which needs to be cleared by coughing.

Poor air quality
Industrial fumes and car pollution will cause irritation of the lining of the throat as will dust. Buildings where central heating dries the air and car exhaust fumes often lead to exposure to dry, poor-quality air. This can

have adverse effects on the throat. Where possible, such situations should be avoided, protection used where appropriate, and the use of a humidifier or ionizer considered.

Smoking

Smoking has serious effects on the lining of the throat. In addition to causing irritation because of the substances contained in the smoke, it causes further drying and promotes mouth breathing. Clearly, it is the main cause of throat cancer.

Anxiety and stress

Stress causes an overall increase in muscle tension and these effects are often noticed in the throat, either as a mild change in the quality of the voice or as a sensation of a tightness or lump in the throat which then leads to constant throat clearing.

Stress also increases acid production in the stomach, which may make the effects of reflux worse.

Coughing and throat clearing

The very act of coughing or clearing the throat can actually cause throat problems to become worse or longer lasting. This occurs as a result of the violent bringing together of the vocal cords, which in itself can cause inflammation in the throat. This can quickly lead to a self-perpetuating condition. Advise your patients to, where possible, try to control the desire to cough or clear the throat. This can be difficult, but swallowing or taking a sip of water will help to take away the sensation. It will also help to moisten the throat and prevent drying.

Infections

URTIs are common, but they can sometimes lead to longer-lasting throat problems. This occurs as a result of excessive coughing and swallowing of mucus, in addition to inflammation of the tissues of the throat. These effects can continue long after the cold itself has gone. Although avoiding infections is not easy, you can advise your patients that if they do get a cold, to: rest, not to try to speak too much, avoid singing or shouting—since this can lead to long-term voice strain—and take plenty of fluids and simple painkillers such as paracetamol.

Drugs

Some drugs can cause a cough or throat problem. ACE inhibitors often cause a side effect of a dry cough. NSAIDs can increase stomach acid and make reflux problems worse.

Gastro-oesophageal reflux disease (GORD) and hiatus hernia

Gastro-oesophageal reflux disease, or GORD, is a common condition. It is caused by changes in the oesophagus and the upper aerodigestive tract due to stomach acid reflux. It is often associated with an incompetent lower oesophageal sphincter or hiatus hernia.

Doctors and patients may not recognize that GORD, a stomach problem, could be responsible for their throat symptoms.

Classical symptoms of GORD
- Heartburn
- Discomfort behind the sternum
- Nausea
- Waterbrash—bitter fluid regurgitation
- Odynophagia—discomfort with hot or cold drinks

ENT symptoms of GORD
- Mucus in the throat
- A feeling of a lump in the throat
- Hoarse voice
- Sore throat on waking

Investigations
Patients with a history of reflux symptoms—such as indigestion, heartburn, and burping—may be treated with a therapeutic trial of a proton pump inhibitor (PPI) for 1 month.

If the GORD recurs, or if the treatment fails completely, patients should be referred for further investigation with an upper GI endoscopy, barium swallow, and 24h pH monitoring.

Conservative treatment
Patients should be advised to:
- Make dietary changes, such as avoiding spicy food, fizzy drinks, and alcohol
- Try to lose weight, if obesity is a problem
- Avoid going to bed within 3h of eating
- Stop smoking
- Prop up the head of the bed on a couple of bricks or blocks

Medical treatment
- Antacids, e.g. Gaviscon®
- H$_2$ antagonists, e.g. ranitidine
- Proton pump inhibitors, e.g. lansoprazole

Surgical treatment
Patients who are resistant to treatment may require anti-reflux surgery, which can be performed laparoscopically.

Neurological causes of swallowing problems

The mechanics of the upper aerodigestive tract are complex. Food, drink, and saliva are directed towards the oesophagus, via the pyriform fossae, while air passes to the lower respiratory tract via the larynx.

The swallowing mechanism is a complex process involving both sensory and motor functions. It is initiated voluntarily but progresses as a dynamic reflex. A neurological condition which affects a patient's motor or sensory function may also cause problems with swallowing.

Common neurological causes of swallowing problems

- CVA (stroke)
- Bulbar palsy
- Motor neurone disease
- Multiple sclerosis
- Tumours of the brainstem
- Cranial nerve lesions, e.g. vagal neuroma
- Systemic neurological conditions, e.g. myasthenia gravis

Investigations

Assessment will involve taking a detailed swallowing history and asking the patient about any coughing or choking attacks, indicating aspiration.

A general neurological examination, and a specific cranial nerve exam, should be done. A CXR may show lower lobe collapse or consolidation if aspiration is present. A video-swallow gives detailed information about the function of the oesophagus (such as delay, pooling, inco-ordination, spasm, etc.). A barium-swallow test may be of limited value because it will only give static pictures.

Treatment

Wherever possible, the patient's underlying condition should be treated, but there will be times when treatment aims to control the symptoms. This could involve:

- Swallowing therapy, as directed by a speech and language therapist
- Dietary modification, such as thickened fluids
- Percutaneous endoscopic gastrostomy (PEG)—a long-term feeding tube
- Cricopharyngeal myotomy—surgical division of the upper oesophageal sphincter muscle
- Vocal cord medialization procedures—where a vocal cord paralysis causes aspiration
- Tracheostomy (📖 see 'The emergency airway', p. 237)
- Tracheal diversion or total laryngectomy (📖 see 'Treatment of laryngeal cancer', p. 226)

Postcricoid web

This is a rare condition and its cause is unknown. An anterior web forms in the lumen at the junction of the pharynx and oesophagus, behind the cricoid cartilage.

Donald Patterson and Adam Brown-Kelly (UK) as well as Henry Plumber and Porter Vinson (USA) describe this condition—their names are frequently used in association with the syndrome.

A postcricoid web is linked with iron deficiency anaemia, and it has the potential to become malignant. Because of this chance of malignancy, endoscopy and a biopsy are recommended. It may also cause dysphagia, and can be seen on a barium swallow.

The web may be dilated and/or disrupted with the help of an endoscope.

Achalasia

This is a rare condition where there is hypertonia in the lower oesophageal sphincter muscle. No increase in pressure is found at endoscopy. Achalasia appears to be due to an abnormality of the parasympathetic nerve supply within the muscles of the oesophagus.

Signs and symptoms
- Progressive dysphagia
- Regurgitation
- Weight loss

Investigations
A barium swallow may suggest achalasia. An endoscopy is needed to exclude an oesophageal tumour, as this can produce similar X-ray appearance and symptoms.

Treatment
- Inhaled amyl nitrate prior to meals—causes relaxation of the sphincter
- Repeated dilatation—stretches the sphincter
- Cardioplasty—surgical enlargement of the sphincter
- Bypass procedures—surgical bypass of the obstruction

Pharyngeal pouch

This is a type of hernia, or pulsion diverticulum, which affects the junction of the pharynx and oesophagus. Elderly males are most often affected.

It is believed to arise as a result of inco-ordination of the swallowing mechanism leading to an increased intraluminal pressure above the closed upper oesophageal sphincter. As a result of this pressure, the pharyngeal mucosa herniates through an anatomical area of weakness, known as 'Killian's dehiscence'—this lies between the two heads of the inferior constrictor muscle (📖 see Fig. 13.2).

Signs and symptoms

- Dysphagia
- Regurgitation of undigested food
- Halitosis
- Gurgling noises in the neck
- A lump in the neck
- Aspiration
- Pneumonia

Investigations

A barium swallow will indicate the diagnosis. A rigid endoscopy must follow to exclude the rare finding of a carcinoma within the pouch. This is sometimes the result of long-term stasis of its contents.

Treatment

Treatment is only necessary if the patient is symptomatic. Endoscopic stapling of the wall which divides the pouch from the oesophagus is the current treatment of choice. Excision, inversion, and suspension of the pouch have been described but are reserved as second-line treatments.

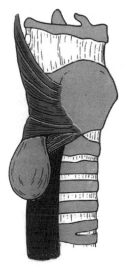

Fig. 13.2 Pharyngeal pouch.

Oesophageal tumours

Benign oesophageal tumours are rare and arise from the local tissue elements, e.g. leiomyoma, adenoma, lipoma.

Malignant oesophageal tumours

The risk factors for a malignant oesophageal tumour include smoking, a high alcohol intake, achalasia, and anaemia. 80% of malignant tumours occur in males who are over 60 years of age. Primary carcinomas are the most common. These carcinomas are squamous and adenocarcinomas. Adenocarcinomas most frequently occur in the lower third of the oesophagus.

The signs and symptoms of a malignant tumour may include weight loss, pain in the throat and/or epigastrium, and progressive dysphagia.

Investigations

- Barium swallow—may show a narrowing or mucosal abnormality suggesting a malignant tumour.
- Endoscopy and biopsy—will confirm the diagnosis.
- CT scan of the chest and abdomen—used to assess extramucosal extent and metastatic spread.

Treatment

- The best chance of a cure is with surgical excision where possible. This may be given with preoperative chemotherapy, and postoperative radiotherapy.
- After the excision, the resulting oesophageal defect will be reconstructed, either with either a stomach pull up, free jejunal grafting, or a myocutaneous flap (📖 see Fig. 13.3).

Where a cure is not possible, palliation may be achieved via:
- Radiotherapy
- Laser debulking of the mass
- Endoscopic stenting
- PEG tube for long-term feeding

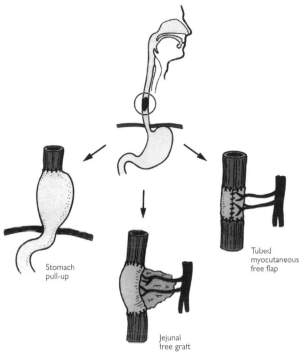

Stomach pull-up

Jejunal free graft

Tubed myocutaneous free flap

Fig. 13.3 Reconstruction.

The neck

Anatomy of the neck

Surface anatomy

Many of the important structures in the neck can be seen or felt on examination. These are:

- The mastoid process (a)
- The clavicular heads (b)
- The sternomastoid muscle (c)
- Trachea (d)
- Cricoid cartilage (e)
- Cricothyroid membrane (f)
- Thyroid prominence (g)
- Hyoid bone (h)
- Carotid bifurcation (i)
- Thyroid gland (j)
- Parotid gland (k)
- Submandibular gland (l)
- Jugulodigastric lymph node (m)

Use Fig. 14.1 to identify the above structures on yourself. It is particularly important to quickly identify the cricothyroid membrane in order to be able to perform an emergency cricothyroidotomy (☐ see 'Cricothyroidotomy', p. 238).

Triangles of the neck

The anterior and posterior triangles of the neck are often referred to in clinical practice and are useful descriptive terms. These triangles may be subdivided as shown in Fig. 14.2a, but the usefulness of the subdivisions is questionable. (This is not to say that an enthusiastic examiner would not be prepared to quiz you on them!)

Deep anatomy

The neck is divided into anatomical compartments by strong fascial layers (☐ see Fig. 14.2b).

- **The posterior compartment**—contains the skeletal muscles of the cervical spine.
- **The anterior compartment**—has additional fascial envelopes containing these important structures:
  - The pretracheal fascia encloses the thyroid gland and binds it to the trachea
  - The carotid sheath encloses the carotid, internal jugular, and vagus nerve

Between these fascial planes lie the parapharyngeal space and the retropharyngeal space. These spaces are clinically relevant because they may become involved in and allow the spread of deep-seated infections or malignancy.

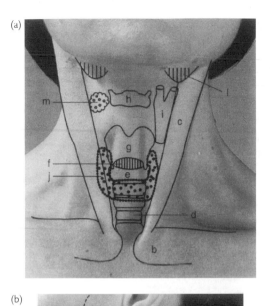

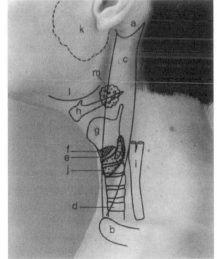

Fig. 14.1 Surface anatomy of the neck.

Lymph node levels

The classification of lymph node levels in the neck are commonly referred to in clinical practice and it is important to have an understanding of them. (📖 See Fig. 14.3.)

Most lymph drainage from the aerodigestive tract is through the deep cervical chain which runs along the internal jugular vein deep to the sternomastoid muscle. It has been discovered that particular anatomical sites drain reliably to particular groups of lymph nodes.

A nodal level system has been devised to simplify the discussion of lymph nodes and to ensure that we are all talking the same language. Essentially this is a naming system which gives a number or level to groups of lymph nodes in a particular area. (📖 See Fig. 14.3 for a diagram of the lymph node levels in the neck.)

This nodal level system is of particular importance when considering the lymphatic spread of ENT cancers. The first group of nodes which a cancer involves is called the 'first echelon nodal level'. For example, the first echelon nodes for tonsil cancer are level 3, from here other nodal levels may be affected, usually levels 2 and 4.

Cancers in other sites may metastasize in different patterns, for example the first echelon nodes from nasopharyngeal cancer tends to be level 5. This concept and model has led to the development of selective neck dissections, e.g. supra-oma-hyoid neck dissections (📖 see 'Neoplastic lymphadenopathy', p. 270).

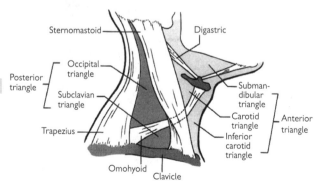

Fig. 14.2a Triangles of the neck.

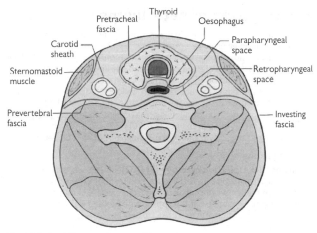

Fig. 14.2b Fascial layers and spaces of the neck.

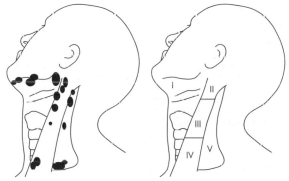

Fig. 14.3 Lymph node levels in the neck.

Investigation of neck lumps

Neck lumps are common. All patients with a neck lump must have an ENT examination to exclude a malignancy.

A full history should be taken, including duration, change in size, smoking history, pain (including referred otalgia), and any intercurrent illness.

A neck lump should be thoroughly examined and the following aspects noted: site, size, shape, texture (smooth or lobulated), position (midline or central), solid or cystic, single or multiple, tender, attached to deep structures, movement on swallowing, movement on tongue protrusion, pulsatile (☐ see 'A lump in the neck', p. 36).

In addition to the above, a full ENT examination should be performed.

Investigations

- **Fine needle aspiration cytology (FNAC)**—is the single most important diagnostic test. It is like a blood test but involves taking cells from the lump rather than blood from a vein. There is no danger of seeding malignant cells if the appropriate method is used (☐ see 'How to perform an FNAC', p. 371).
- **Blood tests**—Where the history suggests an inflammatory mass consider:
  - FBC
  - ESR/CRP
  - Paul–Bunnell/Monospot/IM screen
  - Toxoplasmasis screen
  - HIV test
- **Biopsy**—may be needed if a diagnosis cannot be made. Wherever possible this should be excisional rather than incisional. All but the most trivial neck masses should be biopsied under general anaesthetic.
- **Endoscopy**—cancers of the silent sites of the head and neck may give little or no symptoms themselves but may metastasize to the neck, presenting as a neck mass. Examination of these sites is vital, usually under general anaesthetic, i.e. a panendoscopy, which looks at all the food and breathing passages. The silent sites are:
  - nasopharynx
  - tongue base
  - tonsil
  - vallecula
  - piriform fossa
  - postcricoid region
- Radiology
  - CXR—for malignancy, TB, HIV.
  - Ultrasound scan (USS)—for thyroid, salivary glands. This test is may be useful in children as it is non-invasive and easy, and it can distinguish between a solid or a cystic lump.
  - Spiral CT—rapid acquisition is useful for mobile structures like the larynx and for those patients who find lying flat difficult.
  - MRI—provides excellent soft tissue definition but is degraded by patient movement.

Key point—neck lumps

- FNAC (± USS) is the investigation of choice.
- In expert hands FNAC >80% accurate.
- If the FNAC is non-diagnostic repeat only once and consider excision biopsy and panendoscopy.

Congenital neck remnants

Thyroglossal cysts and fistulae

The thyroid gland develops at the base of the tongue and descends through the tissues of the neck to its final position overlying the trachea. It leaves a tract which runs from the foramen caecum of the tongue to the thyroid gland. This tract curves around the body of the hyoid bone. Thyroglossal cysts and fistulae arise from congenital abnormalities of this process. They are common in teenagers and in young adults.

Signs and symptoms

These may present as a midline, a paramedian swelling, or a discharging sinus. The cyst will rise on tongue protrusion, due to their attachment to the tongue base. (📖 See Fig. 14.4 opposite, and Fig. 15.1, p. 275.)

Treatment

Before surgical excision of the lesion, ensure that there is a normal functioning thyroid gland in its usual position in the neck. Surgical excision, known as Sistrunk's operation, involves removing the lesion plus tissue block between the lesion and the hyoid, plus the mid portion of the hyoid bone and any associated tract passing to the foramen caecum of the tongue. There is a risk of recurrence if less radical procedures are used.

Branchial cysts

These common, benign neck cysts usually appear before the age of 30. They occur at the junction of the upper third and lower two-thirds of the sternomastoid muscle. They often arise following a URTI. They are thought to be caused by degeneration of epithelial inclusions in a lymph node.

Branchial cysts are usually asymptomatic, but they may become painful due to a secondary infection. An FNAC test yields a pus-like aspirate that is rich in cholesterol crystals. The treatment is surgical excision.

In patients over 50 years old, branchial cysts may be confused with metastatic deposits of SCC, which have undergone cystic degeneration. In this group, an FNAC suggesting a branchial cyst should be treated with suspicion.

Branchial fistulae

These arise as a defect in the fusion of branchial clefts. They present as a discharging skin sinus somewhere along the anterior border of the sternomastoid. There is an associated tract, which runs from the skin to the oropharynx, usually ending at the anterior pillar of the tonsil. This tract will pass between the external and internal carotid arteries, in close proximity to cranial nerves X, XI, and XII. Surgical excision of the complete tract, including the tonsil, may be necessary.

Dermoid cysts

These cysts lie anywhere between the chin and the suprasternal notch. They arise from defects in fusion of the midline and are an example of 'inclusion cysts'. They present as painless midline swellings and do not move on swallowing or tongue protrusion. Treatment is via surgical excision.

Cystic hygroma

These are rare, benign lymphangiomas found in neonates and infants. They insinuate themselves between the tissues of the neck and may reach a massive size. They may cause compressive airway symptoms.

Treatment involves securing the airway where necessary, surgical excision can be staged, or injection with sclerosant.

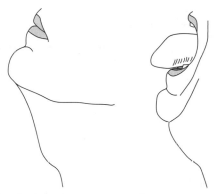

Fig. 14.4 Thyroglossal cysts rise on tongue protrusion.

> ### Key point
>
> **Remember:** Branchial cysts are unusual in middle-aged patients so beware! Metastatic SCC can mimic a branchial cyst on FNAC and imaging and the primary cancer (usually in found in the tonsil) may be completely asymptomatic. Therefore, list for excision as a matter of priority and include a panendoscopy at the same time.

Neck infections

Parapharyngeal abscess

This is a deep-seated infection of the parapharyngeal space (□ see 'Anatomy of the neck', p. 260). It often results from a primary infection in the tonsil, or is an extension from a parapharyngeal abscess (or quinsy) (□ see 'Tonsillitis', p. 194). It is more common in children than in adults.

Signs and symptoms

These include pyrexia, neck swelling deep to the sternomastoid muscle and a patient who seems unwell. There may be trismus, or a reduced range of neck movements. The tonsil and the lateral pharyngeal wall may be pushed medially. Airway compromise is a late and ominous sign.

If the diagnosis is in doubt, a CT scan will often distinguish between lymphadenitis and an abscess.

Treatment

This will involve a high dose of IV broad-spectrum antibiotics (co-amoxiclav), in addition to surgical drainage via a lateral neck approach.

Retropharyngeal abscess

This is a very rare infection of the retropharyngeal space. It is much more common in children and infants than in adults.

Signs and symptoms

An unwell patient, with pyrexia, often with preceding URTI or swallowing difficulty. There may be shortness of breath or stridor, or torticollis—due to prevertebral muscle irritation.

Treatment

A high dose of IV broad-spectrum antibiotics (co-amoxiclav). Where necessary, the airway will be secured and surgical incision and drainage may be performed via the mouth.

Ludwig's angina

This is a rare infection of the submandibular space, it usually occurs as a result of dental infection. It is more common in adults than in children.

Signs and symptoms

These include pyrexia, drooling, trismus, airway compromise due to backward displacement of the tongue. There may be firm thickening of the tissues of the floor of mouth—best appreciated on bimanual palpation.

Treatment

High doses of IV broad-spectrum antibiotics (co-amoxiclav). Secure the airway (try a nasopharyngeal airway first since this will often suffice, but were necessary consider a tracheostomy). Surgical incision is often unsatisfying since little pus may drain away.

Lymph node enlargement

- The majority of neck nodes in children are benign.
- The majority of neck nodes in adults are malignant.
- Neck nodes may be involved secondarily in an infection of any part of the ENT systems.

📖 See 'Lymph node levels', p. 263.

Infective lymphadenopathy

This secondary lymphadenopathy is extremely common in children. An example is jugulodigastric node enlargement during or following tonsillitis. A single node or a group of nodes may be enlarged. There may be tenderness and symptoms related to the primary infection.

Specific infections presenting with lymph node enlargement (primary lymphadenopathy) include:

- Glandular fever
- TB
- Toxoplasmosis
- Brucellosis
- Cat-scratch fever
- HIV

The diagnosis in these cases will often be made following the appropriate screening blood test and CXR. FNAC and even excision biopsy may be needed to exclude malignancy.

Neoplastic lymphadenopathy

Lymphoma

This is a primary malignant tumour of the lymphatic tissues.

Signs and symptoms

Multiple nodes of a rubbery consistency. The patient may or may not experience night sweats, weight loss, axillary or groin nodes, and lethargy.

Investigations

FNAC may be suspicious, but an excision biopsy is often required to confirm the diagnosis and allow for subtyping. A CXR and/or a chest CT scan may be done, or, for staging, a CT scan of the abdomen or pelvis. Bone marrow may be needed for staging.

Treatment

May involve chemotherapy and/or radiotherapy. The patient may need a lymphoma MDT review.

Squamous cell carcinoma

This is a primary mucocutaneous malignancy which commonly spreads to local lymph nodes. It can affect single or multiple nodes.

Signs and symptoms

The patient may have ENT-related symptoms such as a sore throat, a hoarse voice, or otalgia. The nodes may have a firm or hard consistency. The patient may have a history of smoking.

Investigations

These may include FNAC, ENT examination looking for ENT primary carcinoma, a CT or MRI scan of the neck, a CT scan of the chest and/or CXR (metastases), a liver USS (metastases), a panendoscopy, and biopsy.

Where no ENT primary is seen on examination, a rigorous search should be made for a silent tumour. This will usually involve imaging as above with ipsilateral tonsillectomy, biopsy of the tongue base, postnasal space, and piriform fossa as a minimum. (📖 See 'Investigation of neck lumps (Endoscopy)', p. 264.)

Remember: all patients with a neck lump MUST have an ENT examination, including laryngoscopy and endoscopy of the postnasal space. This is essential to exclude a small and asymptomatic malignant primary tumour.
REFER NECK LUMPS TO ENT.

Treatment

This depends on the stage, the size, and the site of the primary (📖 see also Box 14.1). Options for treatment include:

Radiotherapy—involves 4–6 weeks of daily treatment with a total dose of 50–60Gy.

Radical neck dissection—involves removing the affected nodes as well as all the other nodal groups and lymph-bearing structures on that side of the neck. This includes the lymph nodes at level 1, 2, 3, 4, and 5, the internal jugular vein (IJV), the sternomastoid muscle, and the accessory nerve.

Modified radical neck dissection—takes all the nodal levels (1, 2, 3, 4, 5) but preserves one or all of the IJV, the sternomastoid, and the accessory nerve.

Selective neck dissection—instead of all the nodal groups being removed, those groups thought to be at most risk are selectively dissected and removed. All other structures are preserved.

Box 14.1 **N staging of the neck**	
N1	A single node <3cm
N2a	A single node >3cm but <6cm
N2b	>1 ipsilateral node <6cm
N2c	Bilateral or contralateral nodes <6cm
N3	Any node >6cm

Neck hernias

Pharyngeal pouch
📖 See Chapter 13, p. 254.

Laryngocoele
This is caused by expansion of the saccule of the larynx. The saccule is a blind-ending sac arising from the anterior end of the laryngeal ventricle (📖 see Fig. 12.3, p. 215). A laryngocoele is an air-filled herniation of this structure. This can expand, and either remains within the laryngeal framework (internal laryngocoele), or part of it may extend outside the larynx (external laryngocoele). It escapes through a point of weakness in the thyrohyoid membrane.

There is a rare association with a laryngeal cancer of the saccule, and all patients should have this area examined and biopsied.

There is little evidence to support the supposition that this condition is more frequent in trumpet players and glass-blowers.

Signs and symptoms
- Lump in the neck which may vary in size
- Hoarseness
- A feeling of something in the throat FOSIT
- Swallowing difficulties
- Airway problems

If the laryngocoele becomes infected and full of pus (laryngopyocoele) then it may rapidly increase in size and cause additional pain.

The thyroid

Embryology and anatomy of the thyroid

Thyroid problems are frequent topics in both undergraduate and post-graduate exams. It is therefore well worth investing some time in understanding the thyroid.

Embryology of the thyroid

The thyroid begins its development at the foramen caecum at the base of the tongue. The foramen caecum lies at the junction of the anterior two-thirds and the posterior third of the tongue in the midline (□ see Fig. 15.1).

The thyroid descends through the tissues of the neck and comes to rest overlying the trachea. This descent leaves a tract behind it—this can be the source of pathology in later life (e.g. thyroglossal cysts—□ see 'Congenital neck remnants', p. 266).

Anatomy of the thyroid

The thyroid gland is surrounded by pretracheal fascia and is bound tightly to the trachea and to the larynx. This means the gland moves upwards during swallowing. The recurrent laryngeal nerves (branches of the vagus) lie very close to the posterior aspect of the thyroid lobes. These nerves have ascended from the mediastinum in the tracheo-oesophageal grooves and they are at risk in thyroid operations. They may become involved in thyroid malignancy—in cases of malignancy a patient will most often present with a weak and breathy hoarse voice.

The thyroid gland has a very rich blood supply—trauma or surgery to the gland can lead to impressive haemorrhage into the neck.

The parathyroid glands—important in calcium metabolism—lie embedded on the posterior aspect of the thyroid lobes.

> **Key points—thyroid-related swellings**
>
> - Thyroid masses move on swallowing.
> - Thyroglossal cysts move on tongue protrusion (□ see 'Congenital neck remnants', p. 266).

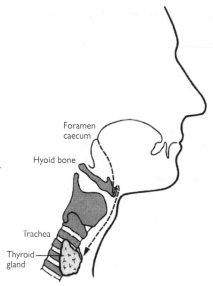

Fig. 15.1 Embryology of the thyroid gland.

Thyroid enlargement (goitre)

Goitre simply means an enlargement of the thyroid gland. It is not in itself a diagnosis. Both physiological and pathological conditions may cause a goitre.

Simple goitre

This is a diffuse enlargement of the thyroid and may result from iodine deficiency. Diffuse enlargement of the gland also occurs in Graves' disease.

Multinodular goitre

This benign goitre is the commonest thyroid problem. It is caused by episodic periods of thyroid hypofunction and subsequent thyroid-stimulating hormone hypersecretion which leads to hyperplasia of the gland. This is followed by involution of the gland. Prolonged periods of hyperplasia and involution are thought to be responsible for the nodular enlargement of the gland found in a multinodular goitre.

A finding of a single nodular enlargement of the thyroid raises the question of malignancy. This should be managed as described (🕮 see Fig. 15.2).

Treatment

A partial thyroidectomy may be necessary but only in a patient with one or all of the following signs:

• Pressure symptoms in the neck
• Dysphagia
• Airway compression
• Cosmetic deformity

Graves' disease

This is an autoimmune condition where antibodies are produced that mimic the effect of thyroid-stimulating hormone (TSH). A hyperthyroid state develops and there is often a smooth goitre. The patient's eye signs may be most impressive (the actor Marti Feldman had this condition). (🕮 See 'Thyroid investigations', p. 280) for eye signs in Graves' disease.

Treatment

Hormonal manipulation with carbimazole. Surgery to correct the proptosis may be achieved via a transnasal orbital decompression. Here, the medial wall of the bony orbit is removed to allow the orbital contents to herniate into the nasal cavity.

Hashimoto's thyroiditis

This is an autoimmune condition where there is often hyperthyroidism and where many patients develop a goitre. Thyroxine replacements may be necessary. Patients with this condition have an increased risk of developing a thyroid lymphoma.

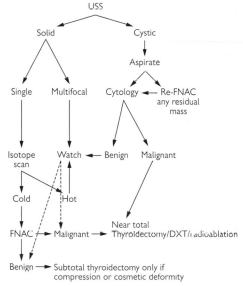

Fig. 13.2 Management of a thyroid lump.

Thyroid neoplasia

Thyroid tumours may arise from either the follicular cells or the supporting cells found in the normal gland. They are quite common and each of these tumours has its own particular characteristics (📖 see Fig. 15.3). Papillary and follicular adenocarcinomas are frequently referred to as 'differentiated thyroid tumours'.

Follicular cell neoplasms

- Papillary adenocarcinoma
- Follicular adenocarcinoma
- Anaplastic adenocarcinoma

Supporting cell neoplasms

- Medullary carcinoma

Papillary adenocarcinoma

These usually affect adults aged 40–50 years. There are usually multiple tumours within the gland. 60% of affected patients have involved neck nodes.

If the disease is limited to the gland, 90% of patients will survive 10 years or more. If the disease has spread to involve the neck nodes, 60% of patients will survive 10 years or more.

Treatment

Involves a near-total thyroidectomy, plus a neck dissection where there are involved nodes. Postoperative radio-iodine may be given to ablate any viable thyroid tissue or tumour left behind after the surgery. After surgery, patients will need lifelong thyroid replacement at TSH suppressing doses.

Follicular adenocarcinoma

It usually affects adults aged 50–60 years. There is a well-defined capsule enclosing the tumour and it spreads via the bloodstream. Up to 30% of patients will have distant metastases at presentation, and hence the prognosis is less good than in papillary adenocarcinoma.

Treatment

As above for papillary adenocarcinoma.

Anaplastic thyroid carcinoma

This condition occurs in adults over 70 years of age, and is more common in women. It involves rapid enlargement of the thyroid gland and pain. The patient will have airway, voice, or swallowing problems due to direct involvement of the trachea, larynx, or oesophagus.

The prognosis is very poor: 92% of patients with this condition will die within 1 year, even with treatment.

Medullary carcinoma

This arises from the parafollicular C cells (or calcitonin-secreting cells). The patient's serum calcitonin level is raised while their serum calcium level remains normal. Neck metastases are present in up to 30% of patients.

Treatment

Involves a near-total thyroidectomy and radiotherapy.

Benign thyroid adenoma

These can be functioning or non-functioning:

Functioning adenomas

They produce thyroxine and will take up iodine and technetium. They appear bright or 'hot' on isotope scanning. Symptoms of thyrotoxicosis may develop. They are rarely malignant.

Treatment is usually medical via thyroid suppressing drugs, but may be treated surgically via excision. Radiotherapy and ablation may be required.

Non-functioning adenomas

These adenomas do not take up iodine. They appear 'cold' on isotope scanning. 10–20% will be malignant. Treatment will be via a surgical excision.

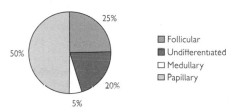

Fig. 15.3 Distribution of thyroid tumours.

Thyroid investigations

Before performing any special investigations look for signs of abnormal thyroid function. Classic signs are given Table 15.1.

Table 15.1 Classic signs of abnormal thyroid function

Hyperthyroidism	Hypothyroidism
Irritability	Mental slowness
Heat intolerance	Cold intolerance
Insomnia	Hypersomnolence
Sweatiness	Dry skin
Amenorrhoea	Menorrhagia
Weight loss	Weight gain
Diarrhoea	Constipation
Palpitations	Bradycardia
Hyperreflexia	Slow relaxing reflexes
Tremor	Loss of outer third of eyebrow
Atrial fibrillation	Hoarse voice

Graves' disease gives rise to particular 'eye signs'. These include:
- Lid lag
- Exophthalmos
- Ophthalmoplegia
- Lid retraction
- Proptosis
- Chemosis

Blood tests

Thyroid function tests (TFTs)

T4 (thyroxine) and T3 (tri-iodo-thyronine) are both bound to plasma proteins in the blood, but a proportion of both remains unbound and these are physiologically active. Bear this in mind when interpreting these results in conditions where the free-to-bound ratio may be disturbed, e.g. nephrotic syndrome or pregnancy.

Thyroid-stimulating hormone (TSH) controls the production of thyroid hormones via a negative feedback mechanism. TSH is usually raised in hypothyroidism and reduced in hyperthyroidism.

Thyroglobulin

This is the carrier protein for T4. Its levels can be measured directly in the blood. It is most frequently used as a tumour marker for the differentiated thyroid carcinomas.

Calcitonin

This is produced by the medullary C cells of the thyroid. Levels are raised in medullary thyroid carcinomas.

CEA—carcinoembryonic antigen

This is a tumour marker of medullary carcinoma of the thyroid.

Thyroid autoantibodies

Specific thyroid autoantibodies can be identified in Graves' disease and Hashimoto's thyroiditis.

Radioisotope scanning

Radiolabelled [^{123}I]iodine or [^{99}Tc^m]technetium is given to the patient orally. Then radiology is used to assess its subsequent uptake into metabolically active thyroid tissue. A thyroid nodule may take up the marker—it will appear bright or 'hot', or it will fail to accumulate the marker—and it will appear 'cold'.

- 80% of thyroid nodules are 'cold'
- 10–20% of 'cold' nodules are malignant
- 'Hot' nodules are almost always benign

Ultrasound (USS)

This is an excellent investigation to demonstrate the thyroid. It will readily distinguish solid and cystic masses inside the thyroid. Often, a USS will show that what appears clinically as a single nodule is in fact part of a multinodular goitre.

MRI/CT scan

These scans may be helpful in determining the extent of a retrosternal swelling. They may confirm airway distortion or compression from a large goitre or they may demonstrate nodal metastases.

Fine needle aspiration cytology (FNAC)

This test will differentiate solid from cystic masses and may diagnose malignancy. A residual mass noted after cyst aspiration should be tested again by FNA to exclude malignancy. It is difficult to distinguish between follicular adenoma and follicular carcinoma. This difference relies on demonstrating capsular invasion which is impossible on cytological features alone. Formal histology is usually required to confirm this diagnosis.

Treatment of thyroid conditions

Management of a thyroid lump

This is best shown diagrammatically, 📖 see the flow chart in Fig. 15.2.

Hormonal manipulation

Thyroxine

Patients experiencing hypothyroid states and after thyroidectomy may need to take thyroxine for life. Doses of levothyroxine sufficient to suppress the TSH production are given in well-differentiated thyroid cancers to reduce tumour growth since these tumours are also TSH-driven.

Carbimazole or propylthiouracil

May be given in hyperthyroidism since these inhibit the formation of T3 and T4.

Radioactive ablation

Most well-differentiated thyroid tumours will trap iodine. This ability can be put to therapeutic effect by administering radioactive iodine. The patient is first rendered hypothyroid by thyroidectomy. The tumour cells then become hungry for iodine and as such will avidly take up the radioactive iodine to their own cytotoxic demise! Radio-iodine therapy can also be used to control a persistent hyperthyroid state.

Thyroid surgery

Thyroid surgery is generally safe and well tolerated by patients.

Hemithyroidectomy

This involves the removal of one thyroid lobe. It is indicated in benign thyroid conditions and as an excisional biopsy procedure where malignancy is suspected but not confirmed.

Total thyroidectomy

This is indicated in thyroid malignancy. Because it increases the risks to the recurrent laryngeal nerves and to the parathyroid glands, some surgeons will perform a near-total thyroidectomy, leaving a small amount of thyroid tissue behind in the area of the recurrent laryngeal nerve.

Risks and complications of thyroid surgery

Some of the most common and important risks of thyroid surgery are given below.

Vocal cord palsy

This is due to recurrent laryngeal nerve damage. Patients will present with a weak and breathy voice. All patients should undergo a vocal cord check preoperatively to document cord mobility before the procedure.

Bilateral vocal cord palsy

This will lead to medialization of the vocal cords resulting in life-threatening airway obstruction. Facilities for re-intubation and tracheostomy must be readily available.

Haematoma

Haematoma after thyroid surgery is another potentially serious complication. This is because the vascular nature of the thyroid can lead to a rapid accumulation of blood in the neck, resulting in compression of the airway. For this reason, all thyroidectomy patients should have stitch/clip removers located at the bedside. If a patient's neck begins to swell rapidly after thyroid surgery, the wound should be re-opened (on the ward if necessary), the clot evacuated, and the airway restored. Once the airway has been secured, the bleeding point can be found and controlled.

Hypocalcaemia

This should be anticipated whenever a total thyroidectomy has been performed. Daily calcium levels should be checked and the patient should be observed for the signs of hypocalcaemia such as:

- Tingling in the hands and feet
- Perioral paraesthesia
- Muscle cramps
- Carpopedal spasm— muscle spasms affecting the hands and feet
- Chvosteck's sign—facial spasm seen on tapping over the facial nerve in the region of the parotid
- Tetany—generalized muscle spasm

As soon as hypocalcaemia is suspected the patient should be given IV calcium gluconate and started on oral replacement therapy.

Sleep-disordered breathing

Sleep physiology

Classification of sleep

REM—20% of sleep time (rapid eye movements seen under closed lids during sleep)
Non-REM—80% of sleep time. Subdivided into stages by EEG activity:
* Stage I—Theta waves. Myoclonic jerks
* Stage II—50% of REM. Sleep spindles and K-complexes
* Stage III—Deep sleep or slow-wave sleep (SWS) characterized by delta waves. Sleep walking, sleep talking, bed wetting and night terrors (stage IV has recently been amalgamated with stage III).

One sleep cycle consists of REM and the three stages of non-REM sleep. It lasts 90 minutes and recurs 3–4 times per sleep.

Causes of altered sleep
* Sleep disordered breathing, e.g. OSAS
* Drugs, e.g. caffeine, energy drinks, amphetamines, cocaine
* Age, i.e. increasing arousals with age
* Sleep pathology:
  * narcolepsy
  * Periodic limb movement disorder (PLMD)
  * Restless leg syndrome (RLS)
  * primary insomnia

Effects of altered sleep
* Excessive daytime sleepiness
* Cardiovascular morbidity and mortality
* Depression
* Increased likelihood of motor vehicle accidents
* Poor work performance

Assessment of sleep-disordered breathing

History

The history of sleep-disordered breathing is often derived from the spouse or partner. It is therefore important that this person attends the consultation. Their observations are an indication only and no substitute for polysomnography. Ask specifically about:

- Snoring—how loud?, every night?, how frequently during the night?
- Apnoeas (breath holding) and their duration
- Limb movements
- Daytime sleepiness (Epworth Sleepiness Score [ESS]—see Epsworth sleepiness questionnaire)
- Weight gain
- Alcohol and drug intake
- Coexisting medical conditions

Examination

- Height and weight to calculate BMI ((height in cm)^2/weight in kg)
- Collar size
- Nose to assess septal deviation, turbinate hypertrophy, rhinitis
- Mouth—Mallampati grade or Friedman Classification System, 📖 see p. 295.
- Mandible—?retrognathic
- Assess craniofacial abnormalities
- Perform nasendoscopy with Muller manoeuvre (nasendoscope is placed at the back of the nose. The patient pinches their nose and takes a breath in with their mouth closed. Collapse can be seen at the level of the palate or tongue base to determine the site of obstruction. Not always reliable.)

The outcome of the consultation

To:

- Exclude a primary sleep disorder that needs evaluation by a specialist sleep physician
- Determine the likely site of obstruction:
  - nasal cavity
  - oropharynx and palate
  - tongue base
  - **or** need for examination under sedation 'sleep nasendoscopy', if uncertain
  - NB there may be more than one site of obstruction in 60% of patients
- Plan further investigations, e.g. a sleep study (particularly if the ESS >12)
- Plan treatment if no further investigations are necessary

Epworth sleepiness questionnaire

Ask the following questions: How likely are you to fall asleep performing these activities?

Score the chances for each situation as:

Never doze	0
Slight chance of dozing	1
Moderate chance of dozing	2
High chance of dozing	3

Sitting and reading
Watching television
Sitting inactive in a public place (e.g. in a theatre)
As a car passenger for an hour without a break
Lying down to rest in the afternoon
Sitting and talking to someone
Sitting quietly after lunch without alcohol
In a car, while stopping for a few minutes in traffic

Total score relates to risk of sleep apnoea
0–10   Normal
10–15   Sleepy
15–20   Risk of apnoea
>20   High risk of OSAS. Suggest to patient they refrain from driving and operating machinery.

Mallampati grading

Classified by the structures seen whilst the patient's mouth is open and their tongue is protruded
- Class I—the soft palate, fauces, uvula, anterior and posterior pillars are visualized
- Class II—the soft palate, fauces, and uvula are visualized
- Class III—the soft palate and base of the uvula are visualized
- Class IV—the soft plate is not visualized

Sleep studies

These studies produce an objective measure of sleep-disordered breathing. At the simplest level the test may represent overnight oximetry. At the other end of the spectrum full polysomnography is performed in a sleep lab and a multitude of variables are measured.

Common parameters measured
- Pulse oximetry to assess oxygen levels
- Nasal airflow
- Chest movements
- Abdominal movements
- ECG heart rate measurement
- EEG measures brain wave activity
- Snoring duration and loudness recording in dB
- EOG measures eye movements

Apnoea hypopnoea index (AHI)

This defines the number of apnoeas and hypnoeas measured in one hour of sleep. Definitions of these parameters vary, but the following are commonly accepted:
- **Apnoea**—cessation of breathing for longer than 10 seconds. (Central apnoea due to neurological problems is not associated with any chest wall movements but obstructive apnoeas are.)
- **Hypopnoea**—decrease in airflow by 30% from baseline and associated with a >4% decrease in oxygen saturations
- AHI <5 normal
- AHI 5–14 mild apnoea
- AHI >30 severe

Sleep study outcome
- Determines whether there is any apnoea
- Determines whether apnoea is due to an obstructive or central cause
- Provides guidance for treatment based on the AHI and the degree of obstruction caused by upper airways resistance

Sleep-disordered breathing spectrum

Sleep-disordered breathing is recognized as a spectrum of problems, ranging from simple snoring to severe obstructive sleep apnoea. Clinical examination combined with sleep study results will help to identify a patient's position on this spectrum

Snoring

This is simply the noise made during sleep. There is no associated sleep disturbance or obstruction seen on the sleep study. ESS <10 and AHI <5.

Snoring often causes marital discord and social embarrassment. Normal laminar airflow through the hypopharynx, oropharynx, and nasal cavity causes no noise. Narrowing of any part of the airway can cause turbulent airflow, which can lead to vibration of tissues in the airway, usually the uvula and soft palate. This is the commonest anatomical origin of the snoring sound.

Upper airway resistance syndrome (UARS)

- Patients snore and experience daytime somnolence
- ESS>10
- No significant apnoeas: AHI <5
- Obstruction causes arousal from sleep before hypoxic change occurs. This leads to changes in the sleep cycle, less REM and non-REM stage III, and less restful sleep

Obstructive sleep apnoea syndrome (OSAS)

- Patients snore and experience marked daytime sleepiness
- ESS >15
- Often markedly obese BMI >30
- Morning headaches
- Memory problems
- Mood alterations
- AHI >5 (the larger the AHI the worse the problem)

Severe OSAS is associated with a risk-independent increase in cardiovascular disease. Mortality and morbidity are increased. There is also a high association with motor vehicle accidents.

Medical treatment

Most patients will have multifactorial disease. Treatment used to be polarized into surgery for snoring and UARS and CPAP for severe OSAS. Nowadays, combination therapy is often necessary.

For all patients
- Lose weight (review by dietician if necessary)
- Stop smoking
- Avoid alcohol
- Treat any associated rhinitis with nasal steroid sprays for at least 6 weeks

Simple snoring
- May require no treatment if partner is happy and severe apnoea has been excluded.
- Sleep positioning can help—try to avoid sleeping on back. Sewing tennis balls into the back of a pyjama top can provide an incentive not to sleep supine.

Oral appliances
There are a variety of designs that:
- Are custom-fit or one size
- Push the mandible forward
- Pull the tongue forward

Upper airway resistance syndrome
As for 'Simple snoring'.
A trial of CPAP may be effective. Often the tolerance of CPAP is related to the degree of daytime sleepiness. The higher the ESS the more likely a patient is to tolerate CPAP. Patients with ESS <12 are often intolerant of CPAP.

Obstructive sleep apnoea syndrome
- CPAP is the mainstay of therapy, and is thought to change the patient's cardiovascular risk if it is effective.
- Surgery is often needed in patients with nasal obstruction and who cannot tolerate CPAP.
- It is important to monitor the patient's tolerance to treatment and the percentage of sleep time that the device is worn. Cardiovascular risk may not change if the patient only wears a CPAP device for part of their sleep.

CPAP therapy

A device delivers a continuous positive airway pressure (CPAP) to prevent collapse of the airway during sleep. This stops the apnoea. Either a sleep study or a self-titrating machine is used to calculate the minimum pressure required to stop the apnoeic episodes.

Bilevel positive airway pressure (BiPAP) is a similar device which has different pressures for inspiration and expiration. It is thought to be better tolerated, especially if high airway pressures are needed.

Complications
- Dry mouth
- Rhinitis and epistaxis

Advantages
- Can be well tolerated
- Relatively cheap compared with surgery
- Can improve daytime somnolence

Disadvantages
- Needs motivation
- Oral side effects, such as excess salivation, muscle spasm, TMJ dysfunction

Surgery for sleep-disordered breathing

Aims of surgery
- Improve tolerance to CPAP
- Increase airway dimensions at specific points to improve airflow
- Stiffen soft tissues to prevent collapse and vibration

Success of surgery
Depends upon:
- BMI
- Correct identification of anatomical sites of obstruction

Predicting success of surgery
- Improved if just a single obstruction site
- Friedman Classification System (opposite) score

Surgical planning
Multiple operations are often required. Simple surgery followed by re-evaluation is the preferred approach. Repeat sleep studies between procedures may help in measuring success.

Surgery by anatomical site
Nose
- Septoplasty
- Reduction of turbinates

Palate and oropharynx
- Tonsillectomy.
- Uvulopalatopharyngoplasty (UPPP)—involves removal of the tonsils, sewing the tonsillar pillars together, and trimming the soft palate. Very painful and can cause a persistent gravel feeling at the back of the mouth.
- Laser-assisted uvulopalatoplasty (LAUP)—here channels are lasered into the soft palate alongside the uvula. Healing causes palatal stiffening.
- Injection snoreplasty—2ml of Fibro-Vein™ is injected submucosally 2cm above the base of the uvula under LA. It stiffens the palate by scarring.
- Somnoplasty™—a radiofrequency probe is inserted into the soft palate under LA. This causes palatal scarring and stiffening.

Tongue base
- Radiofrequency ablation of the tongue base
- Hyoid advancement—this large operation, performed under GA, advances the hyoid to bring the tongue base forward
- Genioglossus advancement
- Bimaxillary advancement—this major surgery is used to correct craniofacial abnormalities when simple surgery or UPPP has failed

Friedman Classification System

The palate position is graded from I–IV, as follows:
- I: The uvula, soft palate, and tonsils/pillars are clearly visible.
- II: The uvula and soft palate are visible, but the tonsils are not.
- III: Only part of the soft palate is visible.
- IV: Only the hard palate is visible.

The tonsil size

This is graded from 0–4, as follows:
- 0+: A previous tonsillectomy has been performed.
- 1+: The tonsils are hidden within the tonsillar pillars.
- 2+: The tonsils extend to the tonsillar pillars.
- 3+: The tonsils extend beyond the pillars but not to the midline.
- 4+: The tonsils extend to the midline.

Surgical staging

- **Stage I** disease includes patients with palate position I or II, tonsil size 3 or 4, and a BMI of less than 40.
- **Stage II** disease includes patients with palate position I or II and tonsil size 0, 1, or 2—**or** palate position III and IV and tonsil size 3 or 4—and a BMI of less than 40.
- **Stage III** disease includes patients with palate position III or IV and tonsil size 0, 1, or 2.

Paediatric ENT problems

Assessing the paediatric patient

Children present several difficulties

- They are small and so is their anatomy
- They are usually unable to give an accurate history
- They have parents who may be very anxious
- Their condition can deteriorate very quickly

Important learning points

- Be able to assess a child in its entirety.
- Gain knowledge of how a child feeds and its daily requirements, especially the total time it takes to feed.
- Become familiar with height and weight charts and the centile ranges which chart a child's physical development.
- Become familiar with the developmental milestones showing a child's speech development (🕮 see Table 17.1).

Shared care

No group of patients demonstrates the principles of shared care better than the paediatric population

Help from paediatricians, midwives, neonatal intensivists, and anaesthetists with special paediatric training is invaluable.

Table 17.1 Language development

Age	Normal language development	Normal speech development	Intelligibility
Infant	Cooing	Non-cry vocalic sounds	
	Babbling	Consonant—vowel syllables with intonation patterns	
1 year	Appearance of first 2–3 words	Omits most final and some initial consonants	Usually no more than 25% intelligible to familiar listener
	Imitates sounds of animals	Substitutes consonants m, w, p, b, k, g, n, t, d, and h for more difficult sounds	
2 years	Uses 2–3-word phrases	Uses above consonants with vowels but inconsistently and with substitution	50–65% of spoken language can be understood
	Has a vocabulary of 250–300 words	Word usage and comprehension develops but comprehension lags behind expressive ability	
	Can put together simple 2–3-word phrases		
	Uses I, me, and you	Can understand much adult communication directed to them	
3 years	Says 4–5-word sentences, with a vocabulary of about 900 words. Uses who, what, and where. Uses plurals, pronouns, and prepositions	Says b, t, d, k, and g, but r and l may be unclear. W is either omitted or substituted. Often repeats self.	75% of communications are intelligible
4–5 years	Vocabulary has increased to about 1500–2100 words. Sentences are complete and most grammar correct	Says f and v. May still have some distortion of r, l, s, z, sh, ch, y, and th	All speech can be understood, although some words may not be perfectly enunciated
5–6 years	Vocabulary of 3000 words	May still distort s, z, ch, sh, and j	

Reproduced with permission from Glasper, McEwing, and Richardson, *Oxford Handbook of Children's and Young Person's Nursing*, page 13, 2007 © Oxford University Press

Neonatal problems

In utero

Occasionally pre-delivery ultrasound scanning can detect congenital problems leading to a planned Caesarean section and possible ENT intervention, for example, cystic hygroma (📖 see 'Congenital neck remnants', p. 266).

The ENT team should be in the theatre, scrubbed and on standby for intubation or tracheostomy if the baby's airway is compromised. Secondary treatment of cystic hygroma is given after further investigation.

Delivery problems

Airway difficulties

Newborn infants are obligate nasal breathers.

Failure to breathe and the development of hypoxia may be related to choanal atresia. The attending paediatrician/anaesthetist may be able to restore breathing with an oral airway.

Bilateral choanal atresia is the likely diagnosis. Failure to pass the nasal suction tube is not always a good sign of atresia.

Placing a metal tongue depressor and watching whether it mists is a good method of measuring nasal airway patency.

Congenital abnormalities

- Microtia
- Branchial cysts or fistulas
- Smaller cystic hygromas
- Haemangiomas

These lesions may all be noticed at birth or during the neonatal examination.

Hearing assessment

Soon all newborn children will be tested for hearing problems in universal newborn hearing programmes. It is important that children who are too sick to be screened are not missed.

Airway problems

Noisy breathing

Many children have periods of noisy breathing. It is **not** normal.

Stertor and stridor are caused by turbulent airflow in the partially compressed airway:

Stertor—is the noise associated with snoring and is due to a supraglottic narrowing of the airway, e.g. enlarged tonsils.

Stridor—is due to narrowing of the airway in and around the glottis and upper airway.

Assessment and examination aim to establish a likely diagnosis and to set parameters for further intervention.

History

- When did it start?
- Related to feeding?
- Position-dependent? Worse on back or front?
- Growth and development
- Neonatal history

Examination

- General examination for birthmarks
- Oral cavity
- Tongue size
- Palate—any clefts?
- Tonsil size
- Intercostal recession
- Tracheal tug
- Stridor—time stridor relative to breathing cycle. Is it inspiratory or expiratory?

Laryngomalacia is the commonest cause of stridor in children. It is usually benign and self-limiting. This is often the presumed diagnosis in children with stridor. (📖 See 'Congenital laryngeal lesions', p. 218.)

Examination under anaesthetic in children less than 12 months of age is associated with an increased mortality.

Indications for microlaryngoscopy and bronchoscopy (MLB)

- Failure to thrive
- Cyanosis
- Prolonged apnoeic episodes

Table 17.2 Different sites of airway obstruction lead to different clinical presentations

	Stridor	Voice	Cough
Nasal/oropharyngeal region	Stertor	Muffled	–
Supraglottis, glottis	Inspiratory	Hoarse	Barking
Subglottis, extrathoracic tracheal	Biphasic	Normal	Brassy
Intrathoracic tracheal, bronchi	Expiratory	Normal	+

Feeding problems

Is this a primary feeding problem or secondary to an airway problem?
  Investigations are usually conducted with the help of a paediatrician and paediatric SALT.

History

- When did it start?
- Regurgitation present?
- Choking?
- Aspiration?
- Weight/height gain?
- Stridor present or absent?

Examination

- Nasal airway—clear or obstructed?
- Mouth and tongue—any enlargement or tongue tie?
- Palate—any clefts present?
- Tonsils—are they enlarged?

Investigation

- Watch bottle or breastfeeding
- Nasal endoscopy to examine larynx and vocal cord movement
- Barium swallow with paediatric SALT in attendance
- Consider examination under GA if no obvious cause and child is failing to thrive

Management

- Nutrition and fluid intake may necessitate NG feeding
- Depends on underlying condition

Snoring and sleep apnoea

This is a common problem in children. Commonest age is from 3–8 years when adenoidal hypertrophy is greatest. The aetiology is different to that in adults.

History from parents
- Mobile phone video often documents episodes
- Apnoeic episodes
- Daytime sleepiness is often not a feature
- Irritability is probably the manifestation of inadequate sleep

Examination
- Nasal obstruction not relieved by vasoconstrictor
- Large tonsils

Sleep studies
- Developmental or syndromic children may have central apnoea as the cause of their snoring and sleep apnoea. Sleep study will show apnoea is not associated with respiratory efforts.
- History of cardiac disease can be associated with central apnoea.

Medical treatment
- Useful for children with obvious rhinitis and hypertrophied turbinates. May also decrease the size of the adenoidal pad.
- Use intranasal steroids, e.g. fluticasone 1 spray into each nostril od for at least 6 weeks.

Surgery
Adenotonsillectomy is usually curative. However, it carries the risk of postoperative haemorrhage and is uncomfortable.

Speech development problems

Speech production

Cognitive ability interacts with the physical method of speech production:

Pulmonary phase—generates constant airflow to the larynx

Laryngeal phase—production of sound occurs via opposition of the vocal cords and mucosal wave of the vocal fold

Oral phase—modification of the laryngeal sound by the tongue, oral cavity, and sinuses

ENT assessment is mandatory in children who are failing to develop speech properly.

The role of the team investigating the child is to identify the barrier to speech development. Often more than one factor can be responsible and may need to be addressed.

Is this part of a global developmental delay?

- Neonatal history
- Developmental landmarks
- Any family history of developmental problems?

Is there a hearing problem?

- Neonatal history
- Any risk factors?
- Familial hearing problems?
- Syndromic child
- Physical examination
- Microtia
- EAC development
- Tympanometry
- Audiology
- Dual pathology

Is there an anatomical impediment to speech?

- Oral cavity
- Tongue tie
- Cleft palate
- Bifid uvula
- Massive tonsils
- Examination of larynx
- Examination under anaesthesia

Treatment

It is important to treat any hearing problem with hearing aids or surgery, e.g. grommets for glue ear. This is particularly important for children with global developmental delay. Any language development is going to be improved by normal hearing.

Common operations

The consent process

General principles

The GMC has issued clear guidelines to assist the consent process. Its recommendations are summarized below:

- Patients must be given sufficient information—in a way that they can understand—to enable them to exercise their right to make informed decisions about their care
- Patients' rights are protected by law
- Effective communication is the key to informed consent

Consent to investigation and treatment

A doctor undertaking a procedure or investigation will need to obtain the patient's consent. If this is impossible, then consent can be obtained by a nominated, suitably trained and qualified person, who understands the risks involved, and who has sufficient knowledge of the proposed investigation or treatment.

It is important that patients make their own decisions about treatment. Ensuring voluntary decision-making involves giving the patient a balanced view of the options and explaining the need for informed consent.

Forms of consent

Consent can be either implied or express.

Implied consent—is when the patient's actions may be, but are not necessarily, an agreement to treatment.

Express consent—is written consent. It must be obtained and documented in the notes when:

- the treatment or procedure is complex, or involves significant risks and/or side effects
- providing clinical care is not the primary purpose of the investigation or examination
- there may be significant consequences for the patient's employment, social or personal life
- the treatment is part of a research programme

In an emergency, when no consent can be obtained, life-saving treatment can be given without consent.

Reviewing consent

Previously obtained consent must be reviewed prior to investigation or treatment, and especially where:

- significant time has elapsed between obtaining consent and the start of treatment
- there have been material changes in the patient's condition, or in any aspects of the proposed treatment plan, which might invalidate the patient's existing consent
- new, potentially relevant information has become available, about the risks of the treatment, for example, or about other treatment options

Giving the patient sufficient information

- Answer questions honestly, accurately, and objectively.
- Give details of the diagnosis, and prognosis, including the likely prognosis if the condition is left untreated.
- Say if there are any uncertainties about the diagnosis, including options for further investigation prior to treatment.
- Give options for treatment or management of the condition, including the option not to treat.
- State the purpose of the proposed investigation or treatment, give details of the procedures or therapies involved, including subsidiary treatment such as methods of pain relief.
- Tell the patient how they should prepare for each procedure and give details of what they might experience during and/or afterwards, including common and serious side effects.
- Explain the likely benefits and the probabilities of success for each option, discuss any serious or frequently occurring risks, including any lifestyle changes which may be necessary as a result of the treatment.
- Say if a proposed treatment is experimental.
- State how and when the patient's condition and any side effects will be monitored or re-assessed.
- Give the name of the doctor who will have overall responsibility for the treatment and, where appropriate, give the names of the senior members of his or her team.
- State whether doctors in training will be involved, and the extent to which students may be involved in an investigation or treatment.
- Remind patients they can change their minds about a decision at any time and that they have the right to seek a second opinion.
- Give details of any costs or charges which the patient may have to meet.

Presenting information to patients

- Where possible, use up-to-date written material, visual and other aids to explain complex aspects of investigation, diagnosis, or treatment.
- Make arrangements to meet particular language and communication needs wherever possible. This could involve translations, independent interpreters, signers, or the patient's representative.
- Where appropriate, discuss with patients the possibility of bringing a relative or friend, or of making a tape recording of the consultation.
- Use accurate data to explain the probabilities of success, the risk of failure, or any harm associated with their treatment options.
- Be considerate when giving distressing information. Give patients information about counselling services and patient support groups.
- Allow patients sufficient time to reflect, before and after making a decision, especially where the information is complex or the risks are serious.
- Where patients have difficulty understanding information, or where there is a lot of information to absorb, provide it in manageable amounts over a length of time, alongside written or other back-up material. You may need to repeat it.
- Involve nursing staff or other members of the healthcare team who may have valuable knowledge of the patient's background or particular concerns. They could help in identifying what risks the patient should be told about.
- If treatment is not to start until some time after consent has been obtained, the patient should be given a clear route for reviewing their decision with the person providing the treatment.

Establishing capacity to make decisions

Fluctuating capacity

Patients who have difficulty retaining information, or are only intermittently competent to make a decision, should be given assistance to reach an informed decision. Record any decision made while the patient is competent, including the key elements of the consultation. Review these decisions at appropriate intervals before treatment starts, to establish that this decision can be relied on.

Mentally incapacitated patients

If patients lack the capacity to make an informed decision, you may carry out an investigation or a treatment that is judged to be in their best interests—including treatment for any mental disorder—provided they comply with it.

Advance statements

Living Wills or Advance Directives must be respected if they are relevant to the current circumstances.

Children and consent

At 16 years old a young person can be treated as an adult and can be presumed to have the capacity to make an informed decision. A child under 16 may have the capacity to make an informed decision, depending on their ability to understand what is involved.

Where a competent child refuses treatment, a person with parental responsibility, or the court, may authorize an investigation or treatment which is in the child's best interests. The position is different in Scotland, where those with parental responsibility cannot authorize procedures a competent child has refused. Legal advice may be helpful on how to deal with such cases.

'Best interests' principle

This involves looking at the following questions:
- Are there any options for treatment or investigation which are clinically indicated?
- Is there any evidence of the patient's previously expressed preferences, including an advance statement?
- What is your own and the healthcare team's knowledge of the patient's background, such as cultural, religious, or employment issues?
- What are the views about the patient's preferences given by a third party who may have knowledge of the patient, for example the patient's partner, family, carer, tutor-dative (Scotland), or a person with parental responsibility?

Which option least restricts the patient's future choices, where more than one option (including non-treatment) seems reasonable in the patient's best interest?

Applying to the court

Application to the court may be needed if a patient's capacity to consent is in doubt or if there are differences of opinion over the patient's best interest. This can occur for non-therapeutic or controversial treatments such as organ donation, sterilization, or turning off life support.

Complications of ear surgery

There are risks with all surgical procedures. The degree of risk is related to both the specific procedure and to the underlying pathology. The patient should be given an indication of the likely risk in a sensitive way, so that they are not frightened into abandoning surgery.

A full explanation of the underlying condition will highlight the risks of leaving an ear disease untreated. Risks should be documented in the case notes and on the consent form.

The list of complications for the CSOM is similar to that of the operation—the untreated disease carries similar risks as the operation. These are:

- Hearing loss—temporary and permanent. Always obtain an audiogram at least within 3 months of surgery, but preferably nearer to surgery and perform pre-op tuning fork tests
- Tinnitus—temporary and permanent
- Vertigo or unsteadiness—temporary and permanent
- Facial nerve palsy—temporary and permanent
- Wound infection
- Need for further surgery
- Formation of mastoid cavity
- Need for ongoing care, e.g. aural toilet for mastoid cavities

Interoperative considerations

These can be avoided by taking precautions, such as always setting up and checking items, such as facial nerve monitors, yourself. The precautions undertaken in theatre, such as the use of a facial nerve monitor, should be recorded on the operation notes. Any interoperative unusual findings or complications should be witnessed and recorded by a senior colleague if available.

Immediate postoperative period

Check for facial nerve palsy in recovery.

Postoperative ward review

Facial nerve function should be checked, along with the eye movements for nystagmus. Weber's tuning fork test should be performed; the patient should localize to the operated ear.

Complications of nasal surgery

Nasal surgery includes a large range of procedures on both the external and the internal nose. Procedures on the sinuses are also included.

Complications of external nose surgery

- Imperfect cosmetic result
- Poor healing of incisions/granuloma and keloid formation
- Bruising
- Ecchymosis
- Need to wear a nasal splint for a week
- Swelling
- Need for packing

Complications of internal nose surgery

- Bleeding and need for packing
- Infection
- Change in nasal shape, e.g. supratip depression with submucus resection (SMR)
- Persistence of nasal blockage for 3 months
- Need for adjunctive medication

Complications of sinus surgery

- Bleeding
- Infection
- Orbital damage
- Optic nerve damage
- CSF leak
- Orbital haematoma

Prevention of complications

Intraoperative considerations

- Good vasoconstriction to maximize vision in operative field and prevent blood loss
- Head-up position to improve venous drainage
- Using preoperative CT scans displayed during surgery to avoid unexpected anatomical variations
- Use of steroids to reduce oedema in rhinoplasty
- Swab samples for infected sinus problems

Postoperative problems

- Observe for bleeding—repack if necessary
- Check for orbital haemorrhage
- Check for visual disturbance

Complications of head and neck surgery

These procedures are often prolonged. They can have high morbidity rates and sometimes mortality.

The patient group is older and the comorbidities associated with heavy smoking and alcohol abuse make the risks even higher.

Major risks

- Death
- Cardiovascular complications
- Myocardial infarction (MI)
- Deep vein thrombosis (DVT)
- Chest infections
- Pulmonary embolism (PE)
- Flap failure

Preoperative considerations

- Prophylactic antibiotics
- Thromboembolic prophylaxis
- Chest physiotherapy
- Preoperative nutrition—involve dietician
- Stopping smoking
- Admit early for assessment and detox if necessary

Postoperative considerations

- Continued thromboembolic prophylaxis and early mobilization
- Antibiotics
- Chest physiotherapy
- Balance between analgesia and respiratory depression
- Early removal of central and peripheral lines
- Removal of urinary catheter
- Tracheostomy care
- Avoidance of pressure sores
- Early action if suspected complication
- Postoperative care on ITU for selected patients
- Nursing protocols and flap observations

Theatre equipment and its correct use

ENT like other branches of surgery has its own special equipment. It does not take long to become familiar with most instruments, particularly those used for common procedures.

Tips to speed the process

Look at the theatre trays during procedures and ask the theatre sister or scrub staff to go over the instruments with you so that they become familiar and you know their names.

Obtain a theatre instrument catalogue or borrow one from theatre to gain extra familiarity.

When performing surgery try to ask for the instruments by name. (Often the same instruments are called different names depending on where you work—this can add to the confusion.) Two instruments warrant special mention:
- The operating microscope
- The ventilating bronchoscope

The operating microscope

The key elements to the use of the microscope depend upon knowing a few simple points:
- Positioning relative to the patient (Fig. 18.1).
- Positioning of the microscope: arm—elbow away.
- Choosing the correct focal length lens. New microscopes have variable focal lengths but older models usually have:
  - 250mm for ear surgery
  - 400mm for laryngeal work; enables use of longer instruments and the microscope can be further away.
- Adjusting the interpupillary distance. (You have to experiment— measure the distance between your own pupils to give optimum stereoscopic vision.)
- The next skill to master is aligning the microscope to see the tympanic membrane. Ear canal, speculum, and microscope objective have all to be aligned to allow for best view.

The ventilating bronchoscope

This instrument causes lots of frustration and angst. It is seldom used regularly outside of specialist paediatric units. There are lots of small parts which often go missing or are misplaced. It is used for the removal of foreign bodies in young children. The procedures are technically and anaesthetically challenging. It is important to practise putting together the instrument and knowing the individual parts so that its use in an emergency is second nature.

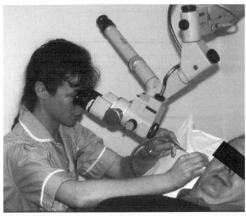

Fig. 18.1 Microscope positioning.

Tonsillectomy

Indications
- Recurrent acute tonsillitis
- Chronic tonsillitis
- Obstructive sleep apnoea syndrome
- Oropharyngeal obstruction
- Following 2 quinsies
- Suspected malignancy
- Diagnosis of variant Creutzfeldt–Jakob disease (CJD)

Preoperative checks
- Confirm that the operation is still needed and examine the ENT system for associated features.
- Discuss the surgery, complications, and the need for time off work or school.

Procedure
- Give the patient a GA and keep them supine with a bolster under their shoulders and their head in a head ring. This position extends head on body. The postnasal space is lower than the oropharynx, so blood collects there.
- Insert a Boyle–Davis gag with Doughty modification for an anaesthetic tube. Place the Draffin bipod to suspend the gag.
- Incise the mucosa over the anterior pillar.
- Remove the tonsil by dissection in the peritonsillar space. Ensure there is adequate tonsil-bed haemostasis.

Postoperative care
- Give appropriate pain relief and encourage the patient to move around. Give food as and when it is tolerated.
- Monitor the patient for blood loss. Major blood loss is obvious, but minor loss in a young child manifests itself as a rising pulse without increasing pain.

Complications
- Primary haemorrhage
- Secondary haemorrhage
- Infection
- Poor pain control

Length of stay
Depends on the unit, the patient may stay in for the day, or overnight.

Discharge advice
Regular analgesia should be taken as the pain often increases around 5–7 days after the operation. Give the patient contact details and advice in case of haemorrhage. They should stay off work or school for 2 weeks and avoid boisterous activity for 2 weeks.

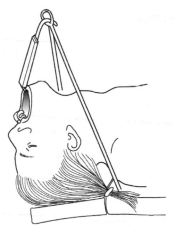

Fig. 18.2 Diagram showing tonsillectomy position.

Adenoidectomy

Indications
The patient may have adenoid problems as a result of, or alongside, glue ear treatment. Removal of the adenoids aids the resolution of glue ear. Patients may experience recurrent adenitis or obstructive sleep apnoea syndrome.

Preoperative checks
- Confirm the diagnosis and the presence of glue with tympanometry.
- Discuss the surgery, complications and need for time off work or school.
- Examine the ENT system for associated features and check the palate for bifid uvula.

Procedure
- Give the patient a general anaesthetic.
- Position them supine with their cervical spine straight. If the spine is extended, as in a tonsillectomy position, the vertebral body of C2 is very prominent and can lead to excess bleeding from postnasal space (PNS) after curettage.
- Check for bifid uvula or submucous cleft.
- Insert an adenoid curette through the mouth into the PNS—curette the adenoidal pad.
- Alternatively, the adenoid can be removed under direct vision with suction monopolar diathermy.
- Haemostasis with pressure from a swab placed in the PNS.

Postoperative care
Give the patient analgesia and observe them for primary haemorrhage.

Complications
- Primary haemorrhage is rare, at less than 1%. If it is uncontrolled it needs a PNS pack, sedation, and an ITU stay for very young children.
- A hypernasal voice (called 'rhinolalia aperta') may occur if there is a defect in the soft palate.
- Subtle malformations such as submucous cleft can be easy to miss and should be looked for before performing an adenoidectomy.

Length of stay
An adenoidectomy is usually a daycase, with the patient discharged after 4 hours, unless it is performed with a tonsillectomy.

Discharge advice
Advise the patient to take regular analgesia and stay off school for 1 week.

Grommet insertion

Indications
The patient may present with glue ear, recurrent acute otitis media, and/or persistent middle ear effusion. They may have Eustachian tube dysfunction. Rarely, the patient may be undergoing hyperbaric oxygen therapy and cannot equalize pressure.

Preoperative checks
- Check that the operation is still required and check tympanometry ± an audiogram.
- Examine the patient's EAC to check access if the operation is being done under local anaesthetic.

Procedure
- Use a local or a general anaesthetic.
- If a local anaesthetic is used, EMLA® cream should be instilled under microscope control. Wait for 60 minutes (send the patient for a cup of tea). Remove the cream by microsuction.
- Using a microscope, insert an ear speculum and identify the antero-inferior segment. Perform a radial myringotomy using a myringotome. Enough fluid is aspirated to allow the grommet to be inserted. The grommet is placed in the myringotomy hole with crocodile forceps, and then adjusted with a needle as required.
- If bleeding occurs, use normal saline drops to help prevent the grommet blocking.

Postoperative care
Use minimal analgesia and give a course of normal saline ear drops—2 drops tds for 5 days   if there is bleeding at the time of insertion.

Complications
This procedure has very few complications. Occasionally, there may be an infective discharge. Treat this with antibiotic or steroid drops for one week.

Length of stay
This procedure is done as a daycase.

Discharge advice
Avoid swimming for 2 weeks. Then use white soft paraffin and cotton wool earplugs with a swimming hat when bathing. Use similar ear plugs for hair washing.

Request a grommet check—community audiogram after 6 weeks—to see if there has been any improvement in hearing.

Septoplasty

Indications

The patient may present with nasal obstruction or may be receiving treatment for epistaxis. As a bent septum can limit surgical access to the sinuses, septoplasty may be needed to correct this before sinus surgery.

Preoperative checks

- Discuss the surgery, complications, and the need for time off work with the patient.
- Examine their ENT system for associated features of rhinitis.
- Discuss their need for possible continuing treatment for associated rhinitis.

Procedure

- Give a general anaesthetic, or a local anaesthetic if the patient is very infirm.
- Lay the patient supine with their head flexed on head ring. The patient's head should be tilted up.
- Infiltrate the local anaesthetic into the septum.
- Approach the septum via a hemitransfixion incision. The mucoperichondrial flaps should be elevated and the cartilage repositioned.
- Resect gross deviations. The 1cm dorsal and anterior struts should be preserved to keep support.
- Suture the incision and pack the nose if necessary.

Postoperative care

Advise the patient to keep their head up and to avoid blowing their nose for 1 week. They should undertake minimal activity for 2 weeks.

Complications

- There may be some bleeding.

Length of stay

- Daycase or overnight stay.

Discharge advice

- Avoid strenuous activity for 2 weeks. A nasal toilet with saline sniffs should be performed four times a day for 2 weeks.

Antral washouts

Indications
Not as widely used as in the past.

The aim of the procedure is to irrigate the maxillary sinus removing any pus, and for:

- Acute sinusitis that has not resolved with antibiotics
- To obtain microbiological cultures where atypical infections are suspected, e.g. in an immunocompromised patient with acute or chronic sinusitis
- As part of another procedure, e.g. clearing the maxillary sinus whilst performing drainage of a periorbital abscess

Preoperative checks
- Discuss the procedure and complications with the patient.
- Confirm the diagnosis on a CT scan.
- Make sure the patient is not on anticoagulants.

Procedure
Perform the procedure under general or local anaesthesia.

- For local anaesthesia, instil 6 sprays of lidocaine with phenylphrine spray into the nostril on the side of the procedure. Sit the patient on an examination chair with their head supported. Alternatively, place the patient on a couch with the backrest raised to at least 45°.
- Soak a cotton wool pledget in 1ml of 5% cocaine solution and insert underneath the inferior turbinate (lidocaine with phenylphrine be used as an alternative and is essential for patients with known cardiac problems.) Leave the patient for at least 6min for the anaesthetic to take effect.
- Remove the pledget. Using a headlight and Thudichum's speculum, insert a Tilly–Lichtwitz trocar and cannula into the nose underneath the inferior turbinate. It will come to rest at the apex of the bony insertion of the turbinate about 2cm from the nostril.
- Align the trocar and cannula with the ear on the ipsilateral side. Gentle pressure breaches the thin medial wall of the maxillary sinus. Advance the cannula and remove the trocar.
- Attach a 10cm syringe containing 5ml of sterile normal saline to the cannula. Aspiration can reveal pus and air. Send any aspirated pus for culture to the first.
- If air is not obtained on aspiration the sinus is probably completely occluded at the natural ostium. Insert a second cannula parallel to the first. Irrigate 200ml of saline through one cannula; the saline then extrudes either into the nose via the natural ostium or back out of the second cannula. Ask the patient to hold a bowl under their chin to catch the flush. Whilst irrigating, observe the cheek and eye for any swelling—suggesting misplacement of the cannula. Once the sinus is clear, stop the irrigation.

Postoperative care
Patients should be advised to undertake minimal activity for 2 weeks.

Complications

There may be some bleeding from the nose. Cheek swelling or orbital haematoma is rare and suggests misplacement of the irrigating catheter outside of the maxillary sinus.

Length of stay

- Daycase or outpatient procedure.

Discharge advice

- Avoid strenuous activity for 2 weeks. Give antibiotic treatment depending on microbiological culture results.

Functional endoscopic sinus surgery (FESS)

Indications
- Chronic rhinosinusitis
- Acute rhinosinusitis
- Complications of rhinosinusitis, e.g. periorbital abscess

Preoperative checks
- Discuss the surgery, complications and the need for time off work with the patient.
- Examine their ENT system for associated features of rhinitis.
- Discuss their need for possible continuing treatment for associated rhinitis.
- Make sure that there is a recent CT scan.

Procedure
Usually performed under GA.
- Place the patient supine in a reverse Trendelenburg tilt of 30°.
- Prepare the nose with Moffitt's solution (2ml of 5% cocaine solution, 1mg of adrenaline and 7ml of 8.4% sodium bicarbonate). Moffitt's solution provides excellent analgesia and vasoconstrictor properties. However, using controlled drugs and the risk of rare but serious cardiac problems must be weighed up by departments. Alternatively, use lidocaine with phenylphrine—6 sprays into each nostril.

The procedure uses endoscopes and special instruments to improve sinus drainage. It usually involves the following basic steps:
- Uncinectomy—removal of the uncinate process
- Middle meatal antrostomy—enlarging the natural maxillary drainage pathway
- Bulla ethmoidalis opening—removal of a prominent anterior ethmoidal bulge which narrows the drainage pathway
- Anterior ethmoidectomy—removal of cells and diseased mucosa of the anterior ethmoid region
- Posterior ethmoidectomy, sphenoidotomy, and opening of the frontal recess (superior drainage pathway of the frontal sinus)—may be performed
- Packs can be inserted, but are best avoided unless excessive bleeding is not controlled by bipolar diathermy coagulation.

Postoperative care
Advise the patient to keep their head up and to avoid blowing their nose for 1 week. They should undertake minimal activity for 2 weeks.

Complications
- Epistaxis—common
- Periorbital haematoma—usually caused by damage to the anterior ethmoidal artery—rare but needs urgent evacuation

- CSF leak—rare but can predispose to meningitis. Clear watery discharge and postoperative headache
- Optic nerve damage—rare

Length of stay

- Daycase or overnight stay.

Discharge advice

- Advise the patient to avoid strenuous activity for 2 weeks.
- Nasal douche with normal saline drops—10ml tds to both nostrils for 2 weeks.
- Prescribe antibiotics—erythromycin 500mg qds for 2 weeks.
- Prescribe prednisolone—40mg od for 1 week—if multiple nasal polyps present.

Ward care

Preoperative care

Pre-assessment

The process of pre-assessment has become established. In many units nurse-led, pre-assessment clinics can identify problems ahead of the planned surgery date, thus avoiding costly delays in the operating schedule. These clinics can only run efficiently if there is good communication between the doctor, nurse, and the anaesthetist.

Protocols have been developed to ensure that only appropriate investigations are ordered, to avoid unnecessary expense.

Clerking

- Effective documentation is important for improved care and to fulfil medicolegal requirements.
- The minimum standard is confirmation of the need for the surgery or investigation, an ENT examination, a list of medications with known allergies, and a list of the results from any investigations ordered.
- Documentation of the consent process is usually provided by the consent form, which is kept in the patient's notes.
- The side of surgery must be marked correctly in accordance with your local hospital policy.
- All relevant investigations and their results must be available in the notes, e.g. biopsy results, recent audiogram, scan results, etc.

Investigations

- Any investigations ordered should be based on the protocol, and discussed with the anaesthetist
- The first step is ordering investigations; but most important is finding and documenting the results of the investigations.

Special considerations

Deep vein thrombosis (DVT) prophylaxis

The risk of DVT for all surgical patients should be classified as low/medium/high. This is determined by the length of surgery, the patient's underlying condition and their past thromboembolic history:

Low   Compression stockings
Medium   Compression stockings + LMW heparin + intraoperative compression boots
High   Compression stockings + LMW heparin/pneumatic + intraoperative compression boots

> **Box 19.1 Low molecular weight heparin** (e.g. dalteparin sodium)
>
> | | |
> |---|---|
> | Medium risk | 2500U 1–2h pre-op |
> | | 2500U every 24h until ambulatory |
> | High risk | 2500U 1–2h pre-op |
> | | 5000U every 24h |

Antibiotic prophylaxis

Antibiotics may be given to patients with pre-existing cardiac problems such as valve problems, or for patients who have had major head and neck surgery, to reduce the risk of postoperative infection and fistula formation:
- Cefuroxime 1.5g 8hrly for 5 days
- Metronidazole 500mg PR 8hrly for 5 days

Diabetic patients

Diabetic patients should be placed first on the operating list. Use blood glucose testing strips regularly to monitor their sugar level. Use a sliding-scale insulin regime for insulin-dependent patients until they are eating.

Postoperative care

Documentation

It is important to document the patient's daily progress and ward round instructions. Any important changes during the day should also be documented. Use a system approach for major head and neck patients, e.g. cardiovascular system (CVS)/respiratory system (RS)/nutrition, etc.

Drain care

Monitor drainage for a 24h period. Remove when it has drained less than 30ml in a 24h period. If the drain loses its vacuum or becomes 'devacced', examine the drain position, change the drain bottle for a new one, and consider pressure to the wound or connect the drain to continuous low pressure wall suction.

Nutrition/fluid balance

Involve a dietician for long-term feeding requirements.

Fluid and electrolytes

Calculate 24h maintenance fluid requirements according to the patient's weight:
- 0–10kg   100ml/kg per 24h
- 11–20kg   1000ml + 50ml/kg/24h
- 20kg+   1500ml + 20ml/kg/24h

This volume of fluid requires a composition of 1–2Eq of Na^+ and 0.5mEq K^+ per kg/24h.
- 1 litre N/saline contains 154mEq of Na^+
- 1 litre D/saline contains 77mEq of Na^+

Maintenance is best undertaken with dextrose/saline to avoid sodium overload, plus the addition of 20mmol/L of K^+.
- Properly kept fluid balance charts are essential in order to monitor the patient's fluid input and output.

Calories

Postoperative patients require between 40 and 70kcal (165–292J) per kg per day. Most ENT patients will be able to be fed either via the mouth or via a nasogastric tube—enteral feeding.

Monitoring intake of calories and other vital substances
- Check weight daily
- Keep a food record chart
- Do regular urinalysis for glucose
- Check levels of FBC, calcium, magnesium, phosphate, zinc, LFTs, U+Es as required
- Screen vitamins and trace elements

Box 19.2 How to unblock a blocked nasogastric tube

- Flush with water
- Flush with soda water
- Flush with a 5% sodium bicarbonate solution
- Aspirate the tube with an empty syringe
- Flush the tube with a smaller syringe
- Use Creon® powder with sodium bicarbonate to flush the tube

Care of myocutaneous and free flaps

It is very important to monitor the viability of these flaps accurately. Often patients are nursed on wards which have limited plastic surgery expertise.
- Ask your local plastic surgeon about the postoperative protocol for the care of free flaps.

General principles
- Maintain intravascular volume
- Maintain oxygen-carrying haematocrit but not polycythaemia
- Monitor flap appearance by using a flap chart
- Monitor blood supply, e.g. Doppler flow.

Protocol example
- Keep pulse <100bpm
- Maintain systolic BP >100mmHg
- Keep urine output >35ml/h
- Aim for haemoglobin level of 8.5–10.5g/dl
- If haematocrit <25% give blood
- If haematocrit >35% give colloid

Flap observations
Doppler and colour observations:
- Every 30min for the first 4h, then
- Every hour for the next 48h, then
- Every 2h for the next 48h

Tracheostomy care

The formation of a tracheostomy causes some physiological problems; mainly because it bypasses the nose. The initial requirements of inspired air are humidification, warming, and filtering. After 48h the mucous glands in the trachea hypertrophy and help in this process.

Irritation caused by the tube

- The presence of the tube can cause coughing and excess secretion from the bronchopulmonary tree.
- Regular suction and inner tube cleaning may be needed as often as every 30 minutes in the initial stages.

Securing the tube

The first tube is usually sutured to the skin to prevent dislodgement. Tapes are then applied, unless there is a free flap where the feeding vessels may be occluded.

In the first week after a tracheostomy the tube should be treated very carefully to prevent dislodgement. The tract between the skin and the trachea is poorly developed and tube displacement during this time could be catastrophic.

Important

Always keep a spare tracheostomy tube and tracheal dilators by the bedside of tracheostomy patients.

Communication with patients and relatives

This is a very important area and one that can cause difficulties. Always treat patients and relatives as you would expect to be treated in a similar situation.

Communication is not just about sitting down and talking with a patient. It can be as informal as saying 'Good morning' in the corridor, or smiling at a patient in a bed near the nurses' station.

Basic principles

- Read the patient's notes thoroughly and be prepared before any formal talk with a patient or their relatives.
- Speak to the nurse looking after the patient for any relevant information.
- Take the nurse with you as a witness or mediator.
- Always speak plainly and try to be honest.

➲ If you are kind and courteous you will have few problems.

Discharge planning

- There is always pressure to discharge patients from the ward with the greatest of haste. Prior planning, often before surgery, can help with this process.
- Nursing staff have good protocols—so liaise with them and seek their advice.

General points

Consideration of the following questions will help in planning effective discharge:

- Is the patient fit to leave—are they orientated, mobile, and pain-free?
- Is the patient's nutritional support catered for?
- Is their wound satisfactory?
- Does the patient need transport?
- Do they have enough medication—both that prescribed in hospital and their regular medication?
- Do any medications need monitoring—such as warfarin?
- Does the patient's GP need to know that the patient is leaving hospital before the discharge letter arrives?
- Is a district nurse required?
- Is outpatient follow-up organized?

Allied health professionals

Who are allied health professionals?

This term covers a number of different professional groups, including:
- Audiologists
- Hearing therapists
- Speech and language therapists (SALT)
- Head and neck specialist nurses
- Dietician
- Aural care nurse

They all have different roles and these are explained in the following pages.

Modern ENT practice has become multidisciplinary, and the involvement of these professionals, alongside members of the medical team, has enhanced patient care significantly.

There are many other personnel who are equally important to patient care, such as physiotherapists and occupational therapists. These are not discussed in this handbook.

➔ It is important to use these professional services properly. Get to know the names of the staff in your department, and find out their particular skills and interests. Try to sit in on their clinics to obtain first-hand knowledge of their areas of expertise.

Communicate with these other professionals and give them the respect that their expertise deserves.

The audiologist

The majority of an audiologist's work is with older people and young children. These age groups comprise the majority of hearing problems. The audiologist has a wide-ranging role, encompassing many aspects of patient care.

The main duties of an audiologist are:
- To assess hearing problems
- To rehabilitate hearing loss with aids
- To assess balance disorders
- To rehabilitate balance disorders
- To give counselling for hearing problems

Many audiologists specialize within the field of audiology. Particular specialties include:
- Paediatric audiology
- Cochlear implant rehabilitation

The role of the audiologist extends to liaising with community peripatetic services. A child of school age will require support in school if their hearing loss has an educational impact. The audiologist can provide an effective route of communication between the school and the ENT department.

→ You will need to understand audiological tests and investigations, as they are an important aspect of ENT care. Audiologists are able to offer advice on appropriate tests and their interpretation.

Every practising otolaryngologist should be able to perform an audiogram and a tympanogram. This is important for clinical practice; in particular, for out-of-hours assessment when no audiological staff are available. Watching an experienced audiologist perform an audiogram is a good way to become familiar with the technique.

Common reasons for referral to audiology

- Adult and children's hearing assessment
- Hearing aid provision
- Vestibular testing

The hearing therapist

This profession has evolved from duties previously undertaken in the audiology department. Many hearing therapists are fully trained audiologists.

The duties of a hearing therapist can include:

- Tinnitus counselling (Fig. 20.1)
- Auditory training
- Counselling for people with hearing impairment
- Supportive counselling for families
- Providing lip-reading advice

The hearing therapist can spend a considerable amount of time with each patient, which allows for an in-depth discussion of a person's difficulties. This can help to improve the quality of life of affected individuals.

Vestibular rehabilitation

Many patients have vestibular dysfunction arising from the causes discussed in Chapter 6. Central compensation for these problems is often complete and unaided. However, a large number of patients have problems in fully compensating for this type of problem. Their symptoms are often compounded by psychological problems caused by the fear of experiencing a vertigo attack. Targeted exercise programmes combined with counselling by a hearing therapist can overcome these difficulties.

Common reasons for referral to hearing therapy

- Tinnitus counselling
- Provision of environmental aids
- Lip-reading

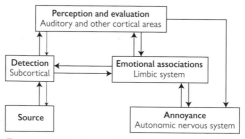

Fig. 20.1 Tinnitus retraining—diagram of model.

Speech and language therapists (SALT)

Speech and language therapists have an important role to play in some ENT conditions. Many patients who are under the care of the ENT department will need specialist input from the SALT team. A major component of their work is dealing with swallowing disorders.

The main duties of a speech and language therapist are:

- Managing communication disorders. This includes:
  - assessing the communication capacity of a patient
  - helping to determine the prognosis for regaining speech
  - determining the patient's need for communication and the aids required
  - providing appropriate advice
- Managing dysphagia. This includes:
  - assessing the type of swallowing problem
  - assessing the risk of aspiration
  - assessing possible interventions

As well as their general duties, the SALT team form part of the MDT managing patients with head and neck cancer and voice disorders.

Voice rehabilitation after laryngectomy

Patients undergoing laryngectomy often fear that they will be unable to communicate after surgery. SALTs may help by introducing patients who have already undergone surgery to demonstrate the range of options for rehabilitation. The options for communication after surgery can include:

- Pen and paper
- Magnetic writing tablets such as Etch-a-sketch™
- Oesophageal speech
- Electric larynx
- Tracheo-oesophageal valves

Common reasons for referral to SALT

- Functional dysphonia
- Assessment of swallowing
- Voice restoration following laryngectomy

The head and neck specialist nurse

This nurse specialist is often the glue which holds the head and neck cancer multidisciplinary team together. The role of the head and neck specialist nurse spans the whole of patient care from diagnosis to preoperative planning to follow-up.

These nurses are uniquely placed to manage patient care; their job flexibility allows them to be active in the community and to extend their care into the home environment. Patients will often view the head and neck nurse as their first point of contact. They are involved early on at the diagnosis stage, up to the patient's final discharge from the clinic.

The main duties of the head and neck specialist nurse are:
- Counselling the patient and their family
- Explaining and giving information on every aspect of care
- Liaising with other members of the MDT
- Assessing the suitability of care options—for example, how the patient might cope with radical surgery
- Mobilizing support from the family and community services

Background of head and neck specialist nurses

These are usually very experienced senior-grade nurses from head and neck specialties. They will have had previous responsibility, usually at ward sister/charge nurse level. They will have a degree-level qualification and experience in head and neck or oncological care.

They will also have good counselling skills and the personality to cope with this demanding job.

Extended roles

A head and neck specialist nurse may also have additional roles:
- Nurse trainer
- Research co-ordinator
- Protocol design
- Independent follow-up clinics

Common reasons for referral to H&N CNS

- All new head and neck cancer patients
- Patients struggling with the consequences of cancer treatments

Dietician

From a nutritional point of view, head and neck cancer patients present a wide variety of challenges. The dietician is an extremely important member of the multidisciplinary team.

The main duties of a dietician are:
- To assess the nutritional status of patients
- To identify specific nutritional concerns
- To plan dietary interventions
- To monitor the patient's response to an intervention

Ongoing research is often an important part of a dietician's role. For example, the role of salicylates in patients with American Society of Anaesthesiologists (ASA) triad and nasal polyps.

Specific problems and areas of work dealt with by a dietician

- Preoperative malnutrition:
  - due to dysphagia from a primary tumour
  - cachexia of malignancy
  - associated alcohol abuse
- Planning preoperative feeding regime
- Planning preoperative route of nutrition, such as PEG/NG tube
- Postoperative nutrition:
  - avoiding re-feeding syndrome
  - managing nutrition in the absence of swallowing
  - non-functioning alimentary tract
  - intolerance to enteral nutrition
  - electrolyte disturbance
- Discharge planning
- Ongoing care, including liaising with community nurses and the patient's family
- Dietary review in outpatients

Box 20.1 Houseman's tip

Dieticians often have essential knowledge of electrolyte replacement and supplementation. This expert knowledge can help in planning nutritional requirements for the optimum care of patients. They will also give advice about the frequency and type of investigations needed to monitor these parameters.

Common reasons for referral to a dietician

- Patients undergoing major treatments for head and neck cancers
- Patients who require dietary modification
- Patients prescribed NG/PEG feeding

Aural care nurse

Aural care nurses provide an important service in the management of ear disorders, and have taken on many aspects of otological care. They are trained to recognize problems in the ear canal and the tympanic membrane. They are also skilled in using the operating microscope. Shared care of patients is important and these nurses should be supervised by, or in close contact with, an otologist.

Areas of expertise of an aural care nurse include:
• Wax removal
• Pre- and postoperative care of patients undergoing ear surgery
• Continued aural care for chronic ear disorders
• Diagnosis and management of otitis externa
• Treatment of mastoid cavity problems

The aural care nurse's efficient management of these conditions—which represent a large amount of clinical otological practice—has led to increased capacity in the outpatient department.

Aural care nurses are graded 1–3 depending on their level of experience. Grade 3 aural care nurses are able to undertake the full range of aural care, from a simple de-wax to the maintenance and cleaning of complex ears with distorted anatomy.

Areas of potential for extending the role of aural care nurses are:
• Direct referral from the GP or A&E
• Nurse prescribing
• Research and development
• Guideline and protocol development

➲ Time spent working with and learning from an aural care nurse can help you develop the skills necessary to perform ear surgery. Experience in using instruments with the operating microscope significantly enhances hand and eye co-ordination.

Common reasons for referral to aural care

• Ear wax requiring microsuction
• Follow-up treatment of otitis externa
• Mastoid cavity patients requiring microsuction
• Postoperative ear care

Common drugs used in ENT

Drugs used in the ear

Topical antibiotics with or without steroids

This group of drugs is widely used for the treatment of otitis externa.

Aminoglycoside group—Sofradex® (framycetin and dexamethasone), Gentamicin, Gentamicin HC (hydrocortisone added)

Indications: Otitis externa

Dosing: 2 drops tds for 10 days

Relative contraindication: Presence of grommet or tympanic membrane perforation due to aminoglycoside ototoxicity in the inner ear. Risk thought to be low in the presence of active infection where the middle-ear mucosa is swollen and the antibiotic is unlikely to reach the inner ear via the round window

Side effects: Sensitivity and allergic reactions. May exacerbate infections

Macrolide group—ciprofloxacin HC

Indications: Otitis externa, necrotizing otitis externa, *Pseudomonas* infection.

Dosing: 2 drops bd to the affected ear for 2 weeks. Longer course in the treatment of necrotizing otitis externa

Side effects: Allergy and sensitivity. No known ototoxicity

Other topical applications

Triadcortyl® cream and ointment (TAC)

Combination antimicrobial and anti-inflammatory agent, contains neomycin, gramicidin, triamcinolone, and nystatin

Indications: Control of mild otitis externa, myringitis, used in aural toilet of mastoid cavities

Dosing: Single application to area of treatment

Side effects: Sensitivity and allergy

Systemic drugs

Betahistine

Action: Increases inner ear blood flow to decrease endolymphatic hydrops

Indications: Prophylaxis against vertigo in patients with Ménière's disease

Contraindications: Peptic ulcer disease and adrenal tumours

Dosing: 16mg tds for at least 6 months. Monitor response with symptom diary

Side effects: Rare and well tolerated. Abdominal bloating and headaches possible

Prochlorperazine

Indications: Control of nausea and vertigo

Dosing: 5mg sub-buccal 8 hourly

Side effects: Extrapyramidal side effects uncommon. Seizures rare

Drugs used in the nose

📖 See Table 9.2, p. 167 for the relative effects of drugs on nasal symptoms

Intranasal steroids

Fluticasone, beclometasone, mometasone

Indications: First-line treatment of rhinitis
Action: Topical anti-inflammatory to reduce chronic inflammation due to allergic and non-allergic causes of rhinitis
Dosing: 2 sprays into each nostril od or bd for at least 6 weeks
Side effects: Nasal crusting and minor epistaxis. Systemic absorbtion not thought to be a problem. Caution in individuals who are taking other topical steroids for asthma or eczema

Oral steroids

Prednisolone

Indications: Treatment of nasal polyposis, pre- and postoperative treatment of patients with polypoid nasal disease
Dosing: 1mg/kg per day for 7 days. Longer courses for patients who have received steroids within the last 3 months will require tapering doses
Side effects: Only associated with prolonged use

Topical antihistamines

Azelastine hydrochloride

Indications: Rhinitis with watery rhinorrhoea
Dosing: 2 sprays into each nostril bd
Side effects: Nasal irritation, headache, and drowsiness

Oral antihistamines

Cetirizine

Action: Selective H_1-receptor antagonist
Indication: Allergic rhinitis and hayfever
Dosing:
- Adults—10mg od
- Children aged 6–18 years—5mg–10mg od
- Children aged 2–6 years—2.5–5mg od
- Children aged 1–2 years—250mcg/kg bd

Side effects: Headache, fatigue, and somnolence rare

Leukotriene inhibitors

Montelukast

Action: Blocks the action of leukotriene D_4 on its receptor
Indications: Patients with Samter's triad or drug-resistant severe rhinosinusitis
Dosing: 10mg od chewable tablet
Side effects: GI disturbance, sleep disorders, increased incidence of Churg–Strauss disease

Drugs used in the treatment of acid reflux

H_2-receptor antagonists—first-line treatment of GORD

Ranitidine
Action: Competitive blocker of histamine at the H_2 receptor. Effective in inhibiting parietal cell acid secretion
Indication: GORD often used in combination with PPI to give better control of nocturnal symptoms
Dosing: 150mg bd up to 300mg
Side effects: Caution in patients with renal and hepatic impairment

Cimetidine
Action: as for ranitidine
Dosing: 400mg bd
Side effects: as for ranitidine

Proton pump inhibitors—second-line treatment of GORD

Omeprazole—20mg bd

Lansoprazole—15–30mg od

Esomeprazole—20–40mg bd
All to be taken at least 30min before food

Action: Directly inhibits the function of the parietal cell proton pump. Reduces acid output and stomach volume
Indication: Failure of first-line treatment in GORD. Severe laryngopharyngeal reflux
Side effects: Minimal

Prokinetic agents

Metoclopramide
Action: Increases lower oesophageal sphincter tone and increases gastric emptying
Indications: Adjunctive treatment for reflux
Dose: 10mg tds

Antacids

Aluminium hydroxide, magnesium hydroxide, sodium bicarbonate, Gaviscon®
Action: Buffer gastric acid by raising pH thus neutralizing stomach acid
Indications: Only used for mild symptoms of dyspepsia. May help symptomatic control with other medications
Dosing: Usually taken with food and just before going to bed
Side effects: Milk alkali syndrome, renal stones, affect absorption of other drugs

ENT manifestations of AIDS

Overview of AIDS

Pathology
- Virus transmitted by sexual contact (70%), needle sharing, and blood products
- Caused by a lentivirus—retrovirus subgroup
- Affinity for CD4 cells
- Enters cells by binding to CD4
- Replicates by using reverse transcriptase
- Viral DNA incorporates into host DNA

Effects
- Direct organ damage
- Decreased efficacy of immune system leading to opportunistic infections

Diagnosis
- Clinical suspicion
- Contact history
- HIV antibodies 95% specific and sensitive

Treatment
- Involve infectious diseases team early. Treatment is determined by specialist team
- Antibiotics
- Antifungals
- Antivirals
- Reverse transcriptase inhibitors, e.g. nucleosidase analogues
- Protease inhibitors. These directly block the production of reverse transcriptase and HIV protease production
- Counselling about the risks of transmission

Specific ENT problems

These are arranged by anatomical site. The treatment of these conditions is often the same as in non-immunocompromised individuals. However, a high index of suspicion for malignancy and atypical infections is necessary. It is common to try to obtain a microbiological specimen and imaging earlier than in standard cases to enable earlier specific antimicrobial treatment and avoid complications.

Skin

Molluscum contagiosum—poxvirus skin lesion produces multiple pedunculated papules approximately 3–4mm. Viral inclusion bodies are seen on microscopy. Approximately 12% of HIV patients have these lesions. They often need treatment with cryotherapy or curettage.

Kaposi's sarcoma—lesions are pathognomonic of HIV/AIDS: red/brown/black papular lesions. The tumour is caused by the human herpesvirus 8. It is a cancer of the lymphatic endothelium rather than a true sarcoma and is highly vascular. Swelling may cause pain. Treatment is palliative. Regression often seen when treating AIDS with antiretrovirals. Treatment is with surgical excision, cryosurgery, or direct interferon injection for isolated lesions; systemic interferon is used for multiple lesions.

Ears

Acute otitis media—has a similar clinical presentation and microbiological cause as in non-immunocompromised patients. Tympanocentesis may be necessary for individuals not responding to first-line antibiotics.

Aural polyps—can be a manifestation of TB or *Pneumocystis carinii* (also known as *Pneumocystis jiroveci*) infection. EAC lesions with granulation can also be caused by these agents. Biopsy under LA and histological and microbiological examination are essential.

Nose and sinuses

Rhinitis—is common in HIV patients. B-cell activation causes an increase in levels of IgE, which cause an increased atopic reaction similar to allergic rhinitis. Treat with fluticasone 2 sprays into each nostril od and cetirizine 10mg od for at least 6 weeks to assess symptom control.

Rhinosinusitis—here, increased rhinitis leads to progressive occlusion of the sinus outflow tract. Hence the patient is more likely to develop sinus symptoms. Failure to respond to topical intranasal steroids and antibiotics, e.g. co-amoxiclav 625mg tds for 1 week, or progressive symptoms, may suggest an atypical organism. CT scan and antral washout may reveal an atypical organism such as a fungus. A scan helps to exclude a tumour.

Oral cavity

Candidiasis—shows as thick white or cream deposits on the mucous membranes. Caused by *Candida* species yeasts. Mucosa is often raised and inflamed. Culture needed for accurate identification. Treatment is with nystatin oral suspension (100 000 units/ml) 4–6mls qds for 2 weeks.

Hairy leukoplakia (30% prevalence in HIV +ve)—is a non-painful white lesion on the lateral border of the tongue. It can be flat or have feathery appearance ('hairy' is misnomer). It is not premalignant and does not need active treatment other than for cosmesis.

Kaposi's sarcoma—as per skin. 95% affect the palate.

Tonsillar hypertrophy—is often due to EBV or CMV infection.

Neck

Lymphadenopathy—can be caused by TB/CMV or acute bacterial infection. FNAC, ultrasound scanning, CT scan, and open biopsy can help determine pathology and plan treatment.

Parotitis—presents with acute pain and parotid enlargement with fever in immunocompromised patients, especially in those with poor oral hygiene. It is due to bacterial infection of the parotid. Treatment with IV antibiotics, e.g. cefuroxime 1g 8–hourly, can be effective. Lack of improvement in 24–48h necessitates CT scanning to exclude an abscess.

Chronic enlargement may be due to tumour, e.g. Burkitt's lymphoma or Kaposi's sarcoma.

Parotid cysts—here, a CT scan may show multiple benign lymphoepithelial cysts. These can be treated with multiple aspirations or parotidectomy (but this carries a risk for facial nerve damage).

Practical procedures

How to cauterize the nose

Always ensure that you have performed adequate first aid steps before attempting to pack or cauterize the nose (📖 see 'Epistaxis', p. 374).

Procedure

- Apply one or two cotton buds or a dental roll soaked in 1:200 000 adrenaline or 5% cocaine solution to the area, and apply pressure for at least 2 minutes.
- Silver nitrate sticks may be applied to the bleeding point for one or two seconds at a time. Avoid using this form of cautery if the nose is actively bleeding since the blood will simply wash the chemical away. In addition to being ineffective, this will cause unwanted burns to the lips, nose, or throat. Instead, wait for the vasoconstrictive effects of the cocaine to work, and then apply pressure to the bleeding point. This will nearly always stop the bleeding temporarily before cautery.
- Apply the silver nitrate in a circle starting a few mm from the bleeding point. This will allow any feeding blood vessels to be dealt with prior to cauterizing the main bleeding vessel.
- It may be necessary to reapply the adrenaline- or cocaine-soaked cotton wool to reduce the bleeding between attempts at cautery.
- If the nose is still bleeding, reapply pressure and consider packing the nose.
- Electro- or hot-wire cautery may be used to good effect in experienced hands.

How to pack the nose

NB Always ensure that you have performed adequate first aid steps before attempting to pack or cauterize the nose (🕮 see 'Epistaxis', p. 374).

When packing the nose, the aim is to put pressure on the bleeding vessel and prevent an active haemorrhage, so that the normal thrombotic mechanisms can act. Nasal packs are usually left in place for 24–48h. They must be secured anteriorly to prevent them falling back into the airway. Prophylactic antibiotics are often used. Patients should be admitted and are often lightly sedated. Different methods and materials are used to pack the nose.

Anterior nasal packing

Nasal tampons

The use of nasal tampons is the simplest way to pack the nose (🕮 see Fig. 23.1). They consist of a dry sponge, which is placed into the nasal cavity and then hydrated with water or saline. The sponge then dramatically increases in size, putting pressure on the bleeding area. The nasal tampon should be lubricated with a little antibiotic cream (Naseptin®). The tip of the nose is simply lifted and the tampon slid into the nasal cavity, ensuring that it is passed parallel to the floor of the nose and not towards the top of the head. A little water or saline is then dripped onto the tampon, which is secured by taping the attached string to the face.

BIPP packing

In this procedure, bismuth iodine and paraffin paste is used to impregnate a length of ribbon gauze. This mixture is antiseptic. Some skill and a good light is needed to place this form of nasal pack effectively. Topical analgesia, such as cocaine spray, is essential prior to packing.

Posterior nasal packing

Epistaxis balloon or urinary catheter

A variety of special nasal balloons are available (🕮 see Fig. 23.2). They are easy to insert and are particularly helpful when the bleeding point is posterior. A Foley urinary catheter is also effective. This is passed into the nasopharynx, inflated, and then pulled anteriorly so that it occludes the posterior choana. It is prevented from slipping back into the nasopharynx or mouth by means of a clamp, which is placed at the nasal vestibule. It is important to put some padding between the skin and a clamp to ensure no pressure damage is caused. Additional anterior nasal packs may be inserted as above where needed.

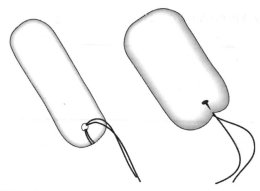

Fig. 23.1 Nasal tampons.

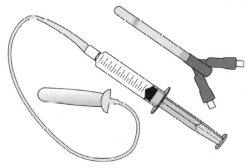

Fig. 23.2 Epistaxis balloons.

How to remove foreign bodies

You will need:
- A good light
- A co-operative patient
- Good equipment

The first attempt will usually be the best tolerated. If you are not confident that you will be able to remove the foreign body, refer to ENT for more experienced help.

Foreign bodies in the ear

Signs and symptoms
- Pain
- Deafness
- Unilateral discharge
- Bleeding
- May be symptomless

Management
- Children will usually require a general anaesthetic unless they are remarkably co-operative.
- Insects may be drowned with olive oil.
- Syringing may be used if you can be certain there is no trauma to the ear canal or drum.
- Use a head lamp or mirror, an operating auroscope or an operating microscope.
- Soft foreign bodies such as cotton wool may be grasped with a pair of crocodile or Tilley's forceps.
- Solid foreign bodies, such as a bead, are best removed by passing a wax hook or Jobson–Horne probe beyond the foreign body and gently pulling towards you.

Refer to senior staff ± GA if:
- Failed attempt
- Unco-operative child
- Suspected trauma to the drum

Foreign bodies in the nose

Signs and symptoms
- Unilateral foul-smelling discharge
- Unilateral nasal obstruction
- Unilateral vestibulitis
- Epistaxis

Management
- An auroscope can easily be used to examine a child's nose.
- Ask the child to blow their nose if they are able.
- Solid foreign bodies such as beads are best removed by passing a wax hook or Jobson–Horne probe beyond the foreign body and gently pulling it towards you. Avoid grasping the object with a pair of forceps, since this may simply push it further back into the nose or airway.
- Soft foreign bodies may be grasped and removed with crocodile or Tilley's forceps.

Refer to senior staff if:
- Failed removal
- Unco-operative child

Foreign bodies in the throat

(📖 See also Chapter 24, 'Oesophageal foreign bodies', p. 384.) The cause is often fish, chicken, or lamb bones.

Signs and symptoms
- Acute onset of symptoms (not days later)
- Constant pricking sensation on every swallow
- Drooling
- Dysphagia
- Localized tenderness in the neck, if above the thyroid cartilage then look carefully in the tongue base and tonsil regions
- Pain on rocking the larynx from side to side
- Soft tissue swelling

Management
- Use a good light to examine the patient.
- Anaesthetize the throat using Xylocaine spray.
- Try feeling for a foreign body (FB) even if you cannot see one in the tonsil or tongue base.
- Flecks of calcification around the thyroid cartilage are common on X-ray.
- Perform an AP and lateral soft tissue X-ray of the neck, looking for foreign bodies at the common sites (◻ see Fig. 23.3). Pay particular attention to the:
  - tonsil
  - tongue base/vallecula
  - posterior pharyngeal wall.
- Tilley's forceps are best for removing foreign bodies in the mouth.
- McGill's intubating forceps may be useful for removing foreign bodies in the tongue base or pharynx.

Refer for endoscopy under GA in case of:
- Airway compromise—**URGENT**
- Failed removal
- Good history but no FB seen
- X-ray evidence of an FB

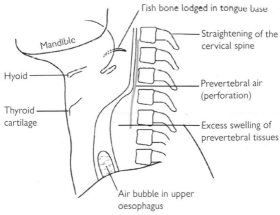

Fig. 23.3 Lateral soft tissues X-ray of the neck.

How to syringe an ear

(📕 See Fig. 23.4.) Check that the patient has no previous history of TM perforation, grommet insertion, middle ear or mastoid surgery.

Procedure

- Warm the water to body temperature
- Pull the pinna up and back
- Use a dedicated ear syringe
- Aim the jet of water towards the roof of the ear canal
- **STOP** if the patient complains of pain

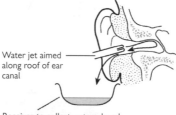

Water jet aimed along roof of ear canal

Receiver to collect water, placed under the ear.
Held in position by the patient

Fig. 23.4 How to syringe an ear.

How to dry mop an ear

A dry mop should be performed in any ear which is discharging, before topical antibiotics and steroid ear drops are instilled.

Procedure

- Tease out a clean piece of cotton wool into a flat sheet.
- Twist this onto a suitable carrier such as an orange stick, a Jobson–Horne probe, or even a clean matchstick (□ see Fig. 23.5).
- Gently rotate the soft end of the mop in the outer ear canal.
- Discard the cotton wool and make a new mop—continue until the wool is returned clean.

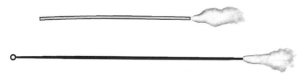

Fig. 23.5 Diagram of an ear mop.

How to instil ear drops

📖 See Fig. 23.6.

Procedure
- Lie the patient down with the affected ear uppermost.
- Straighten the ear canal by pulling the pinna up and back.
- Squeeze in the appropriate number of drops.
- Use a gentle pumping motion with your finger in the outer ear canal.
  This will encourage the drops to penetrate into the deep ear canal.

Consider using an 'otowick'. This is like a preformed sponge and it acts as a reservoir, helping to prevent the drops leaking out of the ear canal. An otowick is particularly useful in otitis externa.

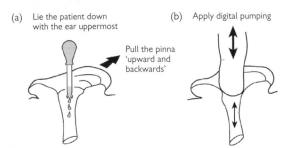

(a) Lie the patient down with the ear uppermost

Pull the pinna 'upward and backwards'

(b) Apply digital pumping

Fig. 23.6 How to instil ear drops.

How to drain a haematoma of the pinna

This usually occurs after direct trauma to the pinna. It is often caused by a sports injury such as boxing or rugby. If left untreated it may leave a permanent deformity such as a 'cauliflower' ear.

Do not neglect the associated head injury which may take priority over the ear injury.

Procedure

- Aspiration may be satisfying, but the collection nearly always reforms, so it is probably best avoided.
- Refer for drainage under sterile conditions.
- Incise the skin of the pinna under local anaesthesia in the helical sulcus (see Fig. 23.7).
- Milk out the haematoma.
- Do not close the wound.
- Apply pressure to the ear to prevent recollection. Either pack the contours of the ear with proflavine or saline-soaked cotton wool, and apply a head bandage. Alternatively, use a through and through mattress suture tied over a bolster or dental roll.
- Give antibiotics.
- Review in 4–5 days.

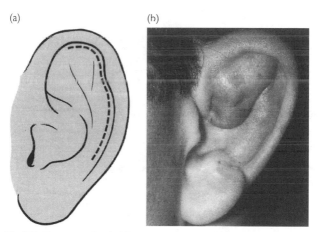

(a)   (h)

Fig. 23.7 Haematoma pinna incision.

How to drain a quinsy

Signs and symptoms
- Sore throat—worse on one side
- Pyrexia
- Trismus
- Drooling
- Fetor
- Peritonsillar swelling
- Displacement of the uvula away from the affected side
  (📖 see Fig. 23.8)

Procedure
- This procedure usually requires admission.
- Rehydrate with IV fluids.
- Give IV antibiotics.
- Spray the throat with lidocaine 10% spray or inject lidocaine into the mucosa
  as shown.
- Lie the patient down.
- Get a good light and a sucker.
- Use a 5ml syringe and a large bore needle or IV cannula to perform 3-point aspiration (📖 see Fig. 23.8).
- Send any pus obtained to microbiology for culture.
- Reserve incision for those cases that recur or fail to resolve within 24h.

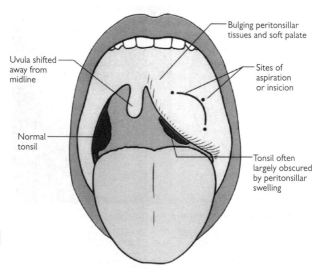

Fig. 23.8 Quinsy/incision/aspiration.

How to perform fine needle aspiration cytology (FNAC)

Procedure

- Lie the patient down.
- Clean the skin with alcohol.
- Fix the lump between your finger and thumb.
- Use a fine needle (blue or orange) attached to a 10ml syringe.
- Pass the needle into the lump.
- Apply suction.
- Move the needle back and forth through the lump using small vibration-type movements—this can prevent contamination by sampling other tissues.
- Make some rotary movements in order to remove a small core of tissue.
- Release the suction.
- Then remove the needle.
- Detach the needle from the syringe and fill it with air.
- Replace the needle and expel the contents onto a microscope slide.
- Remove the needle and repeat as necessary.
- Check the inside of the barrel of the needle for any tissue which may have become lodged there.
- Take a second slide and place it on top of the first, sandwiching the sample between the two.
- Briskly slide the two apart, spreading the sample thinly and evenly.
- Fix and label the slides.

Emergency airway procedures

(📕 See Chapter 12, 'The emergency airway', p. 237)

ENT emergencies

📖 See Chapter 12 for details of:
  The emergency airway
  Stridor
  Epiglottitis
  Supraglottitis
  Croup
  Cricothyroidotomy
  Tracheostomy

📖 See Chapter 23 for details of:
  Quinsy
  ENT foreign bodies
  Auricular haematoma

Epistaxis

Epistaxis, or a nosebleed, is a common problem, which will affect most of us at sometime in our lives. It is usually mild and self-limiting.

Causes of epistaxis

Local causes
- Nose picking
- Idiopathic
- Trauma
- Infection
- Tumours

Systemic causes
- Hypertension
- Anticoagulant drugs
- NSAIDs
- Coagulopathy (haemophilia, leukaemia, disseminated intravascular coagulation [DIC], Von Willebrand's disease)
- Hereditary haemorrhagic telangiectasia (an inherited condition with a weakness of the capillary walls leading to haemangioma formation).

The anterior part of the nasal septum is the most frequent site for bleeding. It has a rich blood supply and a propensity for digital trauma. This part of the nose is known as Little's area (📖 see Fig. 24.1.).

First aid for epistaxis

📖 See Fig. 24.2. The patient should be advised to:
- Lean forward
- Pinch the fleshy part of the nose (not the bridge) for 10 minutes
- Avoid swallowing the blood
- Put an icepack on the nasal bridge
- Suck an ice cube

Resuscitation
- Assess blood loss
- Take the patient's pulse
- Measure the patient's blood pressure
- Gain intravenous access
- Set up an intravenous infusion
- Send blood for full blood count
- Send blood for group and save

📖 See 'How to cauterize/pack the nose', p. 358.

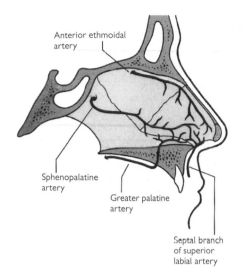

Fig. 24.1 Little's area.

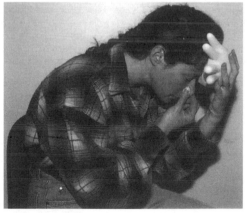

Fig. 24.2 Epistaxis first aid.

Sudden onset hearing loss

Acute sensorineural hearing loss (SNHL) is an ENT emergency. It usually has an acute onset and is sometimes associated with balance disturbance.

Investigations

- Take a full drug history.
- Exclude head or acoustic trauma.
- Check the ear canal to exclude wax.
- Check the eardrum to exclude glue ear.
- Perform tuning fork tests:
  - Weber goes to other ear
  - Rinne AC>BC in affected ear.
- Audiogram confirms hearing loss and no air/bone gap.
- ESR and autoantibodies—may be abnormal if there is an autoimmune cause for the hearing loss.
- MRI to exclude acoustic neuroma—request this as a routine priority unless there is associated neurology.

Management

If the patient presents within 24–48h of onset try empirical treatment as below, but there is little evidence base to support it:

- Admission for bed rest
- Oral steroids (prednisolone 60mg)
- Oral betahistine
- Aciclovir
- Carbogen gas (a mixture of CO_2 and O_2 given for 5min inhalation per waking hour)
- Daily audiograms

If there is any improvement in the hearing at 48 hours, continue with the treatment. If not, discharge on a reducing course of prednisolone and aciclovir.

- Book an outpatient assessment for two weeks' time and re-test the_____ hearing.
- Chase blood and/or MRI results. Consider a hearing aid referral.

Facial palsy or VIIth nerve palsy

Examination of the patient will reveal if the palsy is an upper or lower motor neurone type. The House–Brackmann scoring system is frequently used to record the degree of facial weakness (📖 see Box 24.1).

Upper motor neurone palsy

- Usually as part of a stroke (CVA)
- Forehead spared
- Look for other neurological signs

Lower motor neurone (LMN) palsy

- The entire face is affected, including the forehead
- Taste disturbance may be present as taste fibres run with the chorda tympani branch of the facial nerve

Management

- General neurological and cranial nerve exam—to exclude other neurology.
- Exclude serious head injury—fracture of the temporal bone may lead to disruption of the facial nerve in its intratemporal section.
- Examine the ear—looking for cholesteatoma, haemotympanum, or disruption of the drum or canal.
- Test the hearing.
- Check the parotid for lumps.

Causes of LMN facial palsy

- Bell's palsy
- Ramsay Hunt syndrome
- Acute otitis media
- Cholesteatoma
- CPA tumours such as acoustic neuroma
- Trauma
- Parotid gland malignancies

Bell's palsy—is probably viral in origin, but the diagnosis is made by excluding the other causes shown above. Starting prednisolone (40–60mg) within 48h improves recovery rates. Prognosis is good: 80% of patients fully recover, although returning to full function may take months. As with other causes of facial palsy, the failure of complete eye closure can lead to corneal ulceration, so eye drops or lubricating gel and an eye pad at night may be required. Refer the patient to ophthalmology.

Ramsay Hunt syndrome—this is due to herpes zoster infection of the facial nerve. The features are similar to Bell's palsy with the addition of vesicles on the drum/ear canal/pinna/palate. The prognosis is less good.

Box 24.1 House–Brackmann grading of facial palsy

1 Complete eye closure, normal movement
2 Complete eye closure, mild weakness, barely perceptible
3 Complete eye closure, obvious weakness
4 Incomplete eye closure, obvious weakness
5 Incomplete eye closure, flicker of movement
6 Incomplete eye closure, no movement

Periorbital cellulitis

This is a serious and sight-threatening complication of ethmoidal sinusitis. Treatment should be aimed at the underlying sinus infection, although a combined approach should be followed with input from ENT and ophthalmology.

Presentation
- Preceding URTI
- Swelling of the upper lid and periorbital tissues
- Difficulty opening the eye
- Pain around the eye
- ± Nasal discharge

Investigations
Look for:
- Proptosis
- Pain on eye movement
- Reduced range of eye movement
- Diplopia
- Change in colour vision (red goes first)
- Change in visual acuity

Management
- Have a high index of suspicion. If you are concerned, get a CT scan.
- Get an ophthalmic opinion.
- Take a nasal swab.
- Start IV broad-spectrum antibiotics (e.g. co-amoxiclav).
- Order a CT sinuses coronal (and axial views through the orbits).
- Any compromise in visual acuity/colour vision or suggestion of an intraorbital abscess requires urgent surgical intervention.

If you are treating conservatively, ensure that regular eye observations are performed, as these patients can progress quickly towards blindness.

Fractured nose

Any patient with a fractured nose must have sustained a blow or an injury to the head. Direct trauma to the nose or face is usually from a punch, a clash of heads, or a fall. Brisk but short-lived epistaxis is common afterwards.

In patients with a nasal fracture always consider a head injury and/or cervical spine injury.

Investigations

The diagnosis is made on finding a new deformity to the nose, often with associated epistaxis, facial swelling, and black eyes. Ask the patient if their nose has changed shape as a result of their injury. In the first few days after a nasal injury it can be difficult to assess if there is a bony injury due to the degree of associated soft tissue swelling.

- Try examining the patient from above and behind and looking along the nose from bridge to tip. (📖 See Fig. 24.3.)
- X-rays are not required to make the diagnosis, but may be helpful in excluding other bony facial fractures.
- Exclude a septal haematoma by looking for a boggy swelling of the septum, which will cause total or near-total nasal obstruction. This will require urgent treatment by incision and drainage in theatre.

Treatment

- Treat the head injury appropriately.
- Administer first aid for epistaxis (📖 see 'Epistaxis', p. 374).
- Consider nasal packing if the bleeding continues (📖 see 'How to pack the nose', p. 360).
- Clean and close any overlying skin injuries.
- Make an ENT outpatient appointment for 5–7 days' time. By then, much of the soft tissue swelling will have resolved, allowing assessment of the bony injury. If manipulation under anaesthetic (MUA) is required it can be arranged for 10–14 days after the original injury.

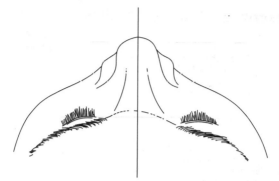

Fig. 24.3 Fractured nose examination (nasal deformity is best appreciated by examining the patient from above ι behind).

Oesophageal foreign bodies

Foreign bodies often impact in the oesophagus. Most pass harmlessly, but hazardous and potentially life-threatening complications may arise. These include: paraoesophageal abscess, mediastinitis, airway obstruction, stricture formation, and tracheo-oesophageal fistula.

Sharp foreign bodies carry a much higher risk of perforation. Take a good history to establish if the patient could have ingested a bone or something similar.

Signs and symptoms

- Immediate onset of symptoms
- Early presentation—hours not days
- Pain—retrosternal or back pain
- A feeling of an obstruction in the throat
- Drooling or spitting out of saliva
- Point tenderness in the neck
- Pain on rocking the laryngeal skeleton from side to side
- Hoarseness—rare
- Stridor—rare but serious

X-ray findings (📖 see Fig. 23.3, p. 365)

- Order a plain soft tissue X-ray of the neck—lateral and AP.
- Not all bones will show on X-ray—so look for soft tissue swelling in addition to a radio-opaque object.
- Look for an air bubble in the upper oesophagus.
- Look for soft tissue swelling of the posterior pharyngeal wall—more than half a vertebral body is abnormal above C4, and more than a whole vertebral body below C4.
- If there is prevertebral air—the oesophagus has been perforated.
- Surgical emphysema is a sign of perforation.
- Loss of the normal cervical spine lordosis suggests inflammation of the prevertebral muscles due to an impacted foreign body or an abscess.

Treatment

Endoscopic removal under GA is often required, and is mandatory if there is any suggestion of a sharp foreign body. If the obstruction is a soft bolus, a short period of observation is appropriate with a trial of a fizzy drink (e.g. Coca-cola®) and IV smooth muscle relaxants (hyoscine butylbromide).

Secondary tonsillar haemorrhage

Bleeding which occurs 5–10 days after a tonsillectomy operation is known as a 'secondary tonsillar haemorrhage'. (A primary haemorrhage is bleeding in the first 24 hours after surgery.) A secondary haemorrhage occurs in less than 10% of cases and may result from an infection of the tonsillar fossa. This condition should not be underestimated.

- Admit the patient.
- Gain intravenous access.
- Give antibiotics and IV fluids.

Occasionally surgical intervention may be needed to achieve haemostasis.

Glossary of ENT terms and eponyms

Key to symbols: 📖 cross-reference; ➲ important; ℘ website

Acoustic neuroma (vestibular Schwannoma): A benign tumour of the eighth cranial nerve

ANCA: Antinuclear cytoplasmic antibody: +ve in Wegener's granulomatosis

Anosmia: Loss of the sense of smell

Antrostomy: An artificially created opening between the maxillary sinus and the nasal cavity

As: Adenoids/adenoidectomy

BAWO: Bilateral antral washouts

BINA: Bilateral intranasal antrostomy

BINP: Bilateral intranasal polypectomy

BNF: *British National Formulary*

BOR: Branchial-oto-renal

BPPV: Benign paroxysmal positional vertigo

BSER: Brainstem-evoked response—an objective test of hearing

Cachosmia: The sensation of an unpleasant odour

Caloric tests: Tests of labyrinthine function

CAT: Combined approach tympanoplasty. A type of mastoid surgery, usually performed for cholesteatoma in which the posterior canal wall is left intact, unlike a modified radical mastoidectomy

CHL: Conductive hearing loss

CJD: Creutzfeldt–Jakob disease

CSOM: Chronic suppurative otitis media

CT: Computed tomography

CXR: Chest X-ray

DL: Direct laryngoscopy

DO: Direct oesophagoscopy

Dohlman's operation: an endoscopic operation on a pharyngeal pouch

DP: Direct pharyngoscopy

EAC: External auditory canal

EAM: External auditory meatus

ENG: Electronystagmography

ENT: Ear, nose, and throat

ESR: Erythrocyte sedimentation rate

EUA: Examination under (general) anaesthesia

EUM: Examination under the microscope—usually of the ears

FBC: Full blood count

FESS: Functional endoscopic sinus surgery

FNAC: Fine needle aspiration cytology

FOSIT: Medical shorthand for a feeling of something in the throat

Free flap: The movement of a piece of tissue (skin ± muscle ± bone) with a supplying artery and vein from one site in the body to another. The blood supply is connected to local blood vessels via a microvascular anastomosis. This is most frequently performed in reconstructing surgical defects following resection of head and neck malignancies

Frey's syndrome: Gustatory sweating, a complication of parotidectomy

GA: General anaesthetic

Globus: A sensation of a lump in the throat, when on examination no lump can be found (see also FOSIT)

Glottis: Another name for the vocal cords

Glue ear: A common cause of conductive hearing loss, due to Eustachian tube dysfunction. The middle ear fills with thick sticky fluid, hence its name. Also known as otitis media with effusion (OME) and secretory otitis media (SOM)

GORD: Gastro-oesophageal reflux disease

Grommet: A ventilation tube placed in the eardrum in the treatment of glue ear also known as 'Gs', 'tympanostomy tubes', or 'vent tubes'

HHT: Haemorrhagic telangiectasia

HIB: *Haemophilus influenzae* type B

HME: Heat and moisture exchanges

HPV: Human papillomavirus

IJV: Internal jugular vein

IV: Intravenous

Ludwig's angina: Infection of the submandibular space

MDT: Multidisciplinary team

ML/microlaryngoscopy: Microscopic surgical examination of the larynx using a suspended rigid laryngoscopy and a microscope

MLB: A diagnostic endoscopy. Microlaryngoscopy and bronchoscopy

MMA: Middle meatal antrostomy. A surgical enlargement of the natural maxillary sinus ostium (📖 See FESS)

MOFIT: Multiple out fracture of the inferior turbinate (See also SMD and TITs)

MRI: Magnetic resonance imaging

MRM: Modified radical mastoidectomy. Mastoid surgery performed for cholesteatoma

MRND: Modified radical neck dissection

MUA: Manipulation under anaesthetic

NARES: Non-allergic rhinitis with eosinophilia

NIHL: Noise-induced hearing loss

od: Once daily

OME: See Glue ear

OSA: Obstructive sleep apnoea

Osteomeatal complex (OMC): The area between the middle turbinate and the lateral nasal wall. The maxillary, frontal, and anterior ethmoid sinuses drain into this area—the final common pathway

Otorrhoea: Ear discharge

Panendoscopy (Pan): Full ENT examination performed under general anaesthetic in order to evaluate/exclude a malignancy of the upper aero-digestive tract

Pec. major: Pectoralis major myocutaneous flap. Frequently used to reconstruct surgical defects in the head and neck region

PEG: Percutaneous endoscopic gastrostomy

PND: Postnasal drip

po: per oral

post-op: Postoperative

PPI: Proton pump inhibitor

pre-op: Preoperative

Presbyacusis: The common hearing loss of old age, high-frequency, bilateral and sensorineural in type

PSCC: Posterior semicircular canal

Quinsy: Paratonsillar abscess

Ramsay Hunt syndrome: Herpes zoster infection of the facial nerve

Reinke's oedema: Benign oedema of the vocal cords caused by smoking

Rhinorrhoea: Nasal discharge

SALT: Speech and language therapist

SCC: Squamous cell carcinoma

Second look: A planned staged operation to ensure that cholesteatoma has not recurred in the mastoid after CAT

Secretory otitis media (SOM): Glue ear

Serous otitis media (SOM): Glue ear

SHO: Senior House Officer

SMD: Submucous diathermy to the inferior turbinates, performed to reduce the nasal obstruction associated with inferior turbinate hypertrophy

SMR: Submucous reception

SNHL: Sensorineural hearing loss

SOHND: Supraomohyoid neck dissection. A type of selective neck dissection

SPR: Specialist Registrar

STIR: Short tau inversion recovery

Ts: Tonsils/tonsillectomy

tds: Three times daily

TITs: Trimming of the inferior turbinates. A surgical procedure performed to reduce the nasal obstruction associated with inferior turbinate hypertrophy, sometimes associated with spectacular haemorrhage!

TM: Tympanic membrane

TMJ: Temporomandibular joint

TSH: Thyroid-stimulating hormone

TTS: Temporary threshold shift

T-tube: Long-term grommet

Tympanometry: The indirect measurement of the middle ear pressure or compliance of the ear drum

Tympanostomy tube: A grommet

URT: Upper respiratory tract

URTI: Upper respiratory tract infection

VOR: Vestibulo-ocular reflux

WS: Waardenburg's syndrome

Index